Dr David Cavan is an experienced consultant endocrinologist with expertise in all areas of diabetes management. He specialises in supporting lifestyle changes to manage and reverse Type 2 diabetes, the use of low carbohydrate and ketogenic diets to promote weight loss and improve health, and the intensive management of Type 1 diabetes.

Also by Dr David Cavan:

How to Reverse Type 2 Diabetes and Prediabetes

Reverse your Diabetes Diet

Take Control of Type 1 Diabetes

The Low-Carb Diabetes Cookbook

Managing Type 2 Diabetes

DR DAVID CAVAN

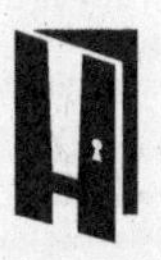

The information in this book may not be suitable for everyone and is not intended to be a substitute for medical advice or medical treatment. You are advised to consult a doctor on any matters relating to your health, and in particular on any matters that may require diagnosis or medical attention. Any use of the information in this book is made on the reader's good judgement after consulting with his or her doctor and is the reader's sole responsibility.

First published in paperback in 2025 by Headline Home
an imprint of Headline Publishing Group

1

Cataloguing in Publication Data is available from the British Library

Paperback ISBN 978 1 0354 1572 4
eISBN 978 1 0354 1573 1

Typeset in Dante by CC Book Production
Printed and bound in Great Britain by Clays Ltd, Elcograf S.p.A.

Headline's policy is to use papers that are natural, renewable and recyclable products and made from wood grown in well-managed forests and other controlled sources. The logging and manufacturing processes are expected to conform to the environmental regulations of the country of origin.

Headline Publishing Group Limited
An Hachette UK Company
Carmelite House
50 Victoria Embankment
London
EC4Y 0DZ

The authorized representative in the EEA is Hachette Ireland,
8 Castlecourt Centre, Dublin 15, D15 XTP3, Ireland
(email: info@hbgi.ie)

www.headline.co.uk
www.hachette.co.uk

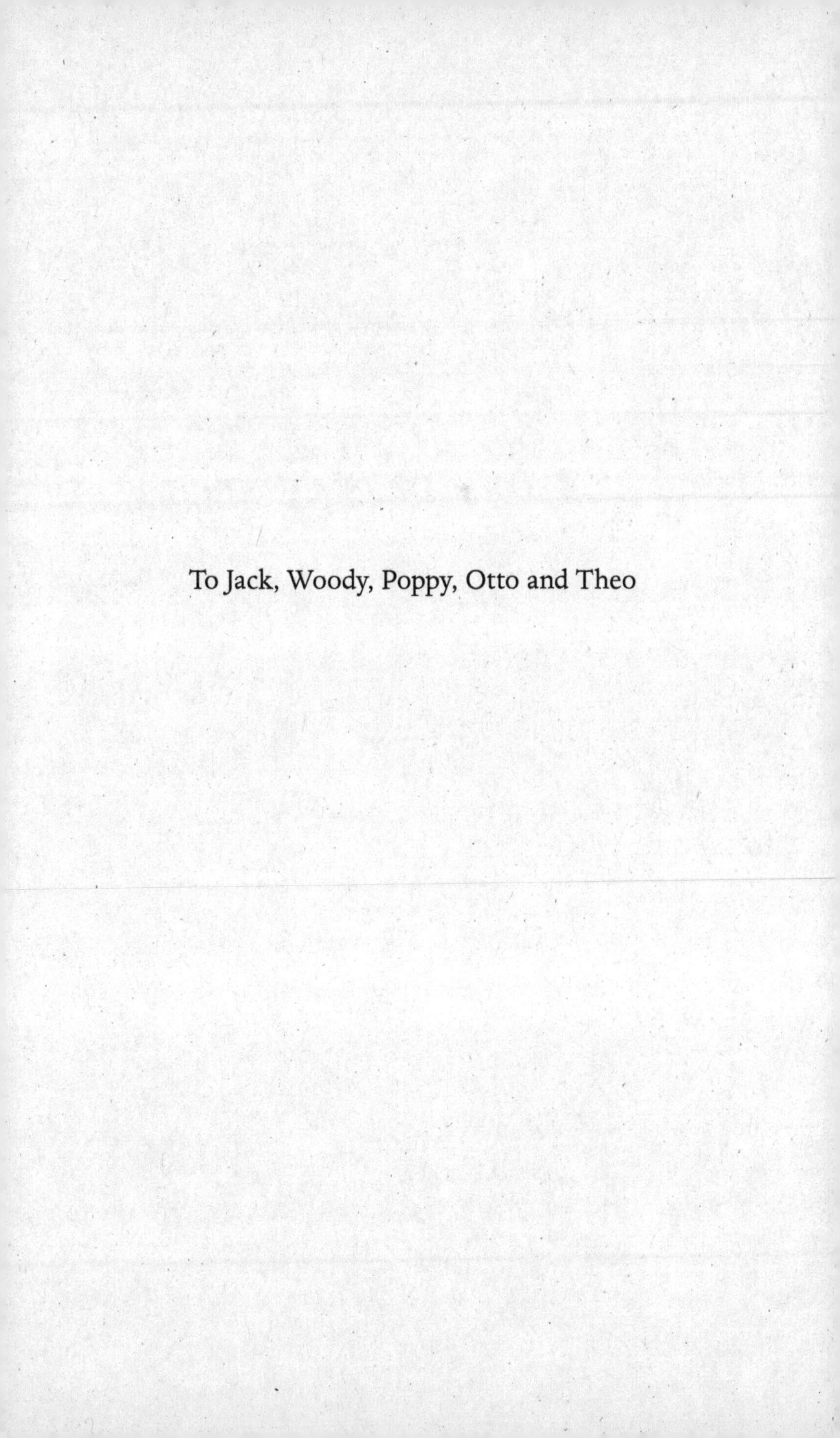

To Jack, Woody, Poppy, Otto and Theo

Contents

Introduction

This may seem a strange thing to say, but now is a really exciting time to have Type 2 diabetes. Why? Because the health prospects of someone with Type 2 diabetes in the 2020s are so very different from just fifteen years ago. Then, the belief was that Type 2 diabetes was a progressive condition that would just get worse over time, requiring more and more medication and, eventually, insulin injections. To make matters worse, despite this treatment, there was the prospect of a host of nasty complications that could cause blindness, kidney failure and amputations. It's easy to see why, for the first half of my thirty-year career as a diabetes specialist, I found Type 2 diabetes thoroughly depressing. And if I found it depressing, how on earth did my patients feel? So what has changed? What has changed is that in 2011, conclusive evidence was published that showed that Type 2 diabetes can be reversed.* The original

* Lim EL, Hollingsworth KG, Taylor E, et al. 'Reversal of type 2 diabetes: normalisation of beta cell function in association with decreased pancreas and liver triacylglycerol.' *Diabetologia*, 2011, 54: 2506–14.

research used a very low-calorie diet for eight weeks but, at the time, I figured that a long-term lower-carbohydrate diet could have a similar effect, and started to recommend this to my patients. Those who followed my advice found that their blood sugar levels reduced and often they needed to reduce their medications. Some of my patients were able to stop insulin injections – something that previously was not thought possible. I have also seen how long-term complications, such as diabetic eye disease, have improved using a low-carbohydrate diet – again, going against the prevailing belief that such complications only get worse over time.

Since then, much research has been published to show how lifestyle changes – or, more specifically, diet changes – can be extremely effective in halting, and even reversing, the diabetes disease process and, in so doing, reducing – not increasing – the need for medication. Not everyone is able to fully reverse their diabetes, but today it is possible to manage Type 2 diabetes by changing your diet and lifestyle, where necessary in conjunction with appropriate medication, to control symptoms and avoid complications, so that you can get on with your life without the fear of inevitably worsening health.

From experience, I know that it is never too late to make changes to improve your health. So, if you have had Type 2 diabetes for many years, there is a real prospect of better health and improved quality of life, possibly requiring less medication. If you have been recently diagnosed, then reversing the condition and achieving remission is a very realistic prospect.

My aim is that this book will provide valuable advice for anyone with Type 2 diabetes, wherever you are on your journey. It contains all the information you need to effectively manage your diabetes, with practical step-by-step advice on the lifestyle changes and medications that will help.

Section 1:

What is Type 2 diabetes?

Chapter 1

A history of diabetes

Its full name is diabetes mellitus, which literally means 'passing honey': untreated diabetes, such as when it's first diagnosed, results in someone passing large amounts of urine containing glucose, and therefore tasting sweet. This is in contrast to a completely different condition called diabetes insipidus, when someone passes large amounts of urine, but it contains no glucose, and so tastes 'insipid'. Thankfully doctors no longer need to taste urine to make these diagnoses!

The first description of diabetes was around 1500 BC in ancient Egypt, as a disease where urine was too plentiful. Accounts from India in 1000 BC reported that the urine was sweet, and that ants and flies were attracted to it. Early physicians thought that diabetes was a disease of the kidneys and bladder. It was noted that diabetes could be inherited (perhaps referring to Type 1 diabetes) or develop because of dietary excess or obesity (Type 2 diabetes). The recommended treatment was exercise. In the seventeenth century it was discovered that the urine of people with diabetes contained sugar, and that diabetes was a disease of the pancreas rather than the kidneys. In 1797, the Scottish military surgeon John Rollo heated the urine of patients until a sugary cake was all that remained. He noted that the volume of the cake increased if the patient ate bread, grains and fruit (high in carbohydrate), but decreased if they ate meat and poultry (low in carbohydrate). He described the case of a patient, Captain Meredith, who adopted a diet low in carbohydrate and high in fat and protein. His weight fell from 224 pounds (105 kg) to 162 pounds (73.5 kg) and his health improved. At the time, diabetes was reported as being relatively rare and associated with wealth.

In 1889 two German physicians from the University of Strasbourg, Joseph von Mering and Oskar Minkowski, removed the pancreas from several dogs. They noticed that this caused the animals to urinate frequently and that the urine contained high levels of sugar, thus establishing a link between the pancreas and diabetes. This was then reversed by transplanting small pieces of the pancreas back into the dog's abdomen.

Piece by piece, the puzzle was being completed, and by the 1920s it had been established that insulin, extracted from animal pancreases and given by injection, led to a fall in blood glucose levels.

What is Type 2 diabetes?

Type 2 diabetes is a condition in which the level of glucose (a type of sugar) in the blood is higher than it should be.

Glucose is used for energy by all types of cells in the body, and it is essential that all parts of the body have a steady supply of glucose. Glucose is obtained from the food we eat: all the carbohydrates (sugars and starches) we eat are broken down into glucose, which is then absorbed into the bloodstream from the gut so it can be carried to the tissues and used as energy. The human body is very efficient at managing glucose, and when everything is working well, we have around 5 grams of glucose in our bloodstream – that is, about a teaspoonful of glucose in 5 litres (8 pints) of blood. This fine-tuned control of the level of glucose in the blood is managed by insulin, which is a hormone that is produced by the pancreas. Insulin works in several ways to ensure that cells get the right amount of glucose at all times:

1. When we eat, any sugar or starch in the food is converted into glucose in the gut, and passes through the gut wall into the bloodstream. The body detects that the glucose level in the blood is rising, and this leads to the pancreas producing additional insulin.

2. This insulin acts on individual cells to allow glucose to enter them. Insulin molecules attach to a receptor on the cell membrane that opens up to allow glucose in. Insulin is often likened to a 'key' that opens the cell's 'door', allowing glucose to enter the cell.
3. Any spare glucose is taken up into the muscles and liver, where it is stored in the form of glycogen. Glycogen in the muscles is then available for later use if the muscles need extra energy (for example, during intensive exercise). Once the glycogen stores are full, any excess glucose is stored in the liver as fat.
4. When we are not eating (for example, overnight), some of the glucose stored in the liver is released into the bloodstream to ensure that enough is available for the body's needs. Insulin acts like a tap that controls this release of glucose from the liver. If the glucose level in the blood drops too low then the pancreas releases less insulin, thus 'opening the tap' to allow more glucose to be released from the liver. On the other hand, if glucose levels rise then more insulin is produced, turning off the tap and slowing the release of glucose from the liver.

The amount of glucose in the blood is expressed as a number of molecules per litre of blood. In the USA and some other countries, a different system is used for measuring glucose levels: there, it is expressed as the number of milligrams of glucose per 100 ml (or decilitre). In a person without diabetes, the normal level of glucose is about 5 mmol/l (millimoles per litre) or 90 mg/dL (milligrams per 100 millilitres). In a person with Type 2 diabetes, the glucose level could be as high as 15 or 20 mmol/l (270–360 mg/dL) – equivalent to two or more dessertspoons of sugar.

Who develops Type 2 diabetes, and how common is it?

Over the past twenty-five years, we have learned a lot about why people develop Type 2 diabetes. In essence, it arises in people who have an unhealthy diet that is high in sugars and refined carbohydrates. It is more common in people who are overweight. Lack of physical activity is also associated with an increased risk of developing Type 2 diabetes. In other words, it is associated with modern lifestyles, and that is why the number of people worldwide with Type 2 diabetes has increased from less than 150 million in 2000 to over 500 million in 2023. In the past, Type 2 diabetes occurred mainly in richer societies, but now it is increasing in almost every country in the world. Tragically, rates in African countries are forecast to more than double in the next twenty years.

How is diabetes diagnosed?

The typical symptoms of diabetes include excessive urination, excessive thirst, tiredness, blurred vision, weight loss, and being susceptible to infections such as thrush. This usually only happens once the glucose level in the blood has reached a high level (above 10 mmol/l or 180 mg/dL) and the kidneys try to get rid of the excess glucose by excreting it in the urine. Glucose in the urine provides an ideal environment for the growth of bacteria and fungi, which leads to urinary infections and thrush (candidiasis). To excrete glucose, the kidneys need to excrete a larger volume of water (otherwise you would be peeing out sugar lumps), and this leads to dehydration, which in turn leads to excessive thirst. High glucose levels in the eyes cause blurred vision.

In many cases of Type 2 diabetes, people are diagnosed with no or only very mild symptoms. This is because diabetes can now be picked up very early from screening blood tests. If someone has had undiagnosed diabetes for some time, blood glucose levels may be high enough for some of these symptoms to occur.

Diabetes is diagnosed by a blood test. This means that, if you have symptoms which you think may be due to diabetes but your blood tests are normal, you do not have diabetes. On the other hand, if your blood tests are diagnostic of diabetes (that is, show that you have diabetes), then you have diabetes, even if you have no symptoms. Nowadays, diabetes is usually diagnosed by the glycated haemoglobin (HbA1c) blood test. It can also be diagnosed by measuring the level of glucose in the blood, either when fasting or after a meal.

Glycated haemoglobin (HbA1c)

When the level of blood glucose is higher than normal, the excess glucose attaches to a number of different molecules in the body. For example, when glucose attaches to the lens of the eye, it can lead to the development of cataracts, or if it attaches to soft tissue in the shoulder it may lead to a frozen shoulder. This process of attachment is called glycation. Red blood cells contain haemoglobin, which is the substance that carries oxygen in blood cells to the different tissues around the body and gives blood its red colour. A small amount of haemoglobin in each blood cell is glycated: just how much will depend on the amount of glucose present in the bloodstream. Red blood cells last for about four months before they are 'recycled', and the amount of glycated haemoglobin in any one cell gradually increases over this time, depending on the level of glucose in the blood. Blood glucose levels change constantly according to food intake and activity levels, so a single measurement is little use in monitoring diabetic control. Glycated haemoglobin, on the other hand, is used to assess glucose levels over a longer period, and for many years has been the 'gold standard' way of assessing diabetic control.

Since 2011, HbA1c has become a recognised method of diagnosing Type 2 diabetes. Measuring it involves a simple blood test that can be taken at any time of day (as it reflects glucose control over the past six to eight weeks). Historically, HbA1c was expressed as the percentage of haemoglobin that was glycated. In 2011, a new system of units was introduced, which expresses the glycated component as a concentration of the total haemoglobin (mmol/mol). In some countries, the older units are still used, and so I will present both units in this book. In people without diabetes, glycated haemoglobin is generally below 42 mmol/mol (6 per cent). This unit of measurement relates to the number of molecules of glycated haemoglobin for every molecule of haemoglobin in the blood.

The World Health Organization (WHO) states that a result between 42 and 48 mmol/mol (6.0 and 6.5 per cent) is indicative of prediabetes, and the UK and many other countries follow this definition. However, the USA and some other countries use slightly different levels, as shown in Table 1.1. A measurement of 48 mmol/mol (6.5 per cent) or above is diagnostic of Type 2 diabetes.

Glycated haemoglobin is also measured to monitor how well diabetes is being controlled, to ensure that the recommended treatment – lifestyle changes and medication – is achieving the desired effect. Generally, a level of 50 mmol/mol (6.7 per cent) or below indicates well-managed diabetes; levels much above 65 mmol/mol (8 per cent) significantly increase your risk of developing diabetes-related complications.

Fasting and random blood glucose level

Sometimes your glucose level will be measured in a blood test taken at any time of day, and this is called a random glucose. This is often the first test that will be done if your GP suspects that you have diabetes, and can be performed at any time of the day after breakfast. If the random glucose is normal, it is unlikely that you have diabetes; however, if the random glucose is in the prediabetes range, then your GP will suggest a fasting glucose taken first thing in the morning. The levels are interpreted as shown in Table 1.1.

Table 1.1. Blood tests used to diagnose prediabetes and Type 2 diabetes.

	Normal	*Prediabetes*	*Diabetes*
Fasting glucose			
mmol/l	Less than 5.5	5.5–7.0	Above 7.0
mg/dL	Less than 100	100–125	Above 125
Random glucose			
mmol/l	Less than 7.8	7.8–11.1	Above 11.1
mg/dL	Less than 140	140–200	Above 200
HbA1c (WHO definition)			
mmol/mol	Less than 42	42–48	Above 48
per cent	Less than 6.0	6.0–6.5	Above 6.5
HbA1c (US definition)			
mmol/mol	Less than 39	39–48	Above 48
per cent	Less than 5.7	5.7–6.5	Above 6.5

What are the types of diabetes?

The currently recognised types of diabetes include:

1. Type 1 diabetes: This usually occurs first in children or young adults. It comes on quite suddenly with marked symptoms such as thirst and weight loss. It is due to the body's immune system destroying the cells in the pancreas that produce insulin. It can only be treated by insulin injections. Blood tests usually show the presence of diabetes-related antibodies.
2. Type 2 diabetes: This usually occurs in later life, and is related to unhealthy food and physical inactivity. It usually comes on more gradually, without any specific symptoms, and is sometimes first diagnosed by a screening blood test. Type 2 diabetes can be controlled by lifestyle changes, principally by modifying diet. Many people are prescribed drugs to control Type 2 diabetes. Until relatively recently, it was thought that most people would eventually need insulin.
3. Prediabetes: This is the stage where blood glucose levels are higher than normal, but not high enough to diagnose Type 2 diabetes. Many people with prediabetes will progress to develop Type 2 diabetes unless they make lifestyle changes.

4. MODY (Maturity-Onset Diabetes of the Young): This is a group of inherited diabetic conditions that are not associated with weight gain. People with MODY usually have a strong family history of diabetes. Although MODY usually presents in childhood, most cases can be controlled with tablets rather than insulin.
5. LADA (Latent Autoimmune Diabetes of Adulthood): This is a type of Type 1 diabetes that occurs in people who are middle-aged or older. Like people with Type 1 diabetes, people with LADA are not overweight and they usually test positive for diabetes-related antibodies; however, the onset is more like Type 2 diabetes. Patients may be treated with tablets first, but within a few years it will become clear they need insulin, and from that time their treatment is the same as for someone with Type 1 diabetes. This 'overlap' between Type 1 and Type 2 diabetes means that, unfortunately, some people are initially given the wrong diagnosis and possibly therefore the wrong treatment – sometimes for many years.
6. Gestational diabetes: This is a condition in which diabetes occurs during pregnancy. It is similar to prediabetes and is usually managed with dietary change at first, although some people do need medication. It usually reverses once the baby is born, but both the

mother and the baby are at increased risk of developing Type 2 diabetes in later life.

7. Secondary diabetes: This arises as a result of other diseases affecting hormones (for example, acromegaly, where there is too much growth hormone, or Cushing's disease, where the body produces too much of the natural steroid hormone, cortisol). These cases generally reverse once the underlying condition has been treated. People who have been treated with high-dose steroid medications for long periods of time for conditions such as asthma can also develop diabetes.
8. Type 3c diabetes: This is a type of secondary diabetes that occurs if other diseases affect the pancreas or if the pancreas has been wholly or partly removed by surgery. It requires treatment with insulin.

While some parts of this book may be helpful to people with other types of diabetes, it is intended for people with pre-diabetes and Type 2 diabetes, to teach them how to manage their condition.

How does Type 2 diabetes develop?

If someone has taken in more energy than they need (via food and drink), their body's cells are full of glucose, so that when insulin opens the cell doors, there is no room for any more glucose to go in. Therefore, the glucose stays in the blood and the level gradually increases. As the glucose level increases, the pancreas produces more insulin to try to push glucose into the cells. They are already full, so instead glucose is taken up into the liver, where it is stored as glycogen. The liver can only store a certain amount of glycogen, so when the glycogen store is full, the excess glucose is converted to fat and stored in the liver. The liver can store almost unlimited amounts of fat: however, as it does so, glucose begins to leak from the glycogen store. Therefore, despite insulin levels being high, the glucose level in the blood increases still further. This is termed insulin resistance. In Type 1 diabetes, the body can no longer produce insulin, but in Type 2 diabetes a patient will often have a high level of insulin, but the body is resistant to its actions: in other words, the insulin can no longer do its job of keeping the glucose level stable. In an attempt to bring the glucose level down, the pancreas produces even more insulin, leading to more fat being stored in the liver, until eventually the body needs to find other storage areas for excess fat, including the pancreas. In the same way that a liver full of fat cannot work properly, a pancreas that is filled with fat can no longer produce insulin. And all the time the glucose in the blood increases until it passes the level for prediabetes and eventually reaches the level to diagnose Type 2 diabetes.

Unlike MODY, Type 2 diabetes is not a genetic condition passed on by genes we inherit from our parents. It is, however, more common in some families than others, and more common in some ethnic groups than others. This suggests that certain genetic traits make it more likely that some people will develop Type 2 diabetes than others. This explains why, while being overweight is associated with an increased risk of Type 2 diabetes, there are some people who are hugely overweight who have completely normal glucose levels – and others who are only a few pounds overweight who have Type 2 diabetes. Type 2 diabetes also tends to occur at a lower body weight in people of Asian or Afro-Caribbean descent than in white Europeans. Some populations have a very high rate of Type 2 diabetes, such as the Pima Indians (a Native American tribe) in Arizona: almost 50 per cent have the condition. However, this is not just due to their genes, as their cousins in the Pima tribe across the border in Mexico have a very low rate of Type 2 diabetes. The difference is that in the USA, the Pima community adopted an unhealthy American lifestyle, whereas in Mexico the Pima continued to follow a healthy, traditional lifestyle – even though, as a country, Mexico has high rates of Type 2 diabetes. Until they changed their lifestyle, the Pima in the US also had very low rates of Type 2 diabetes – as was the case for almost every population across the world. So, certain groups are more susceptible to developing Type 2 diabetes than others – but they will only develop if the conditions are right and they have an unhealthy lifestyle.

The trouble is, this is happening in populations all around the world. When I worked at the International Diabetes Federation (IDF), one of my tasks was to oversee the production of the IDF Diabetes Atlas. This resource is published every two years, and estimates the prevalence of diabetes across the globe.

The first IDF Atlas was produced in 2000, when it estimated that 151 million people had diabetes. By 2021, this figure had increased to 537 million. That means that over just twenty years, the number of people with diabetes increased by more than three-fold. Over the same time, the global population increased by about 28 per cent, from 6.1 billion in 2000 to 7.8 billion in 2020. If the rate of diabetes increased because of the increase in the world population, we would expect the current prevalence to be 193 million, not 537 million. That means over 340 million more people developed diabetes than expected, and over 300 million of those are likely to have developed Type 2 diabetes.

So how has this come about? Could it be the result of an infection? Could it be the result of a new genetic disease? Or could it be the result of something else?

A disease that spreads by infection usually spreads quite rapidly – in the case of Covid-19, over 100 million people developed the disease in the first year. On the other hand, genetic changes take several generations to show their impact, and the diseases that result increase much more slowly. The only possible explanation for this rise in Type 2 diabetes is that people have been affected by something else in their lives that has changed their metabolism.

And that leads to the next question. What has changed in our lives in the past few decades? To help answer this, have a think about everyday life now compared with when you were a child. What has changed about how we live our lives, how we get about, how we communicate with each other and how we work, play and go shopping? Even if you are only thirty, you will be able to remember a time before smartphones, Facebook, online shopping and online banking. If you are sixty, you will remember a time before there were fast-food restaurants and coffee shops on every high street, before freezers and microwaves appeared in the home, before ready meals and takeaways, and when a can of Coke or a packet of crisps was a special treat. You will also remember when many more jobs involved manual labour. If you are eighty, you will remember food rationing after the Second World War, and if you are older than that, you may remember food shortages and hunger.

As a result of these changes, our levels of physical activity have progressively reduced. We spend many more hours sitting down (such as in front of a screen) than any other generation in history. There has also been a massive increase in car ownership: far more of us get around by driving our own car rather than walking or using public transport.

The other major change to our lives has been to our diet. Imagine a household that had neither a freezer nor a microwave. What would that mean for the type of food the inhabitants ate? It would mean no ice cream or frozen ready meals. It would mean no microwave ready meals (which usually contain highly processed ingredients). So, in this imaginary home, meals are much more likely to be prepared from fresh ingredients each day. Up to the 1970s, this was reality, and fast food was a strange American phenomenon, rarely found in Europe. Fast forward fifty years and almost every high street, shopping centre and motorway service station has several fast-food outlets selling highly processed, high-calorie, low-cost foods. For some people, they have become part of their staple diet, rather than an occasional treat.

Finally, our physical environment can aggravate the effect of other changes to our lifestyle, especially for people who live in a 'food desert': this means an area, often in a poorer neighbourhood, where there are no shops that sell healthy foods. Paradoxically, while fresh food is hard to find in such places, fast-food outlets are often very common. Your environment determines what you can eat.

The food industry has also hugely influenced what is available for us to eat. Over the past twenty years these companies have exploited the addictiveness of certain ingredients and adjusted the formulation of their products, precisely to make us want to eat more. Then they market those products with advertising that is designed to make us want to buy the product.

As a result of all these changes, people worldwide have seen massive lifestyle changes – we sit around more, walk less, and eat more highly processed foods. The effect of these changes is that, as a global society, we have gained weight, accumulated excess fat in our internal organs, and set off the metabolic derangements that lead to Type 2 diabetes. As a result, what was a relatively unusual condition just a few decades ago is now reaching epidemic proportions.

Whenever I speak about this process, I always emphasise that, just like every other creature, human beings eat food that is readily available in our environment. That means that if you have developed Type 2 diabetes, IT IS NOT YOUR FAULT. Yes, we can all make choices about which foods to buy, but our choices are distorted by the massive, poorly regulated marketing of the food industry. Its marketing is designed to trigger emotions in us, to influence our choice towards their ultra-processed products (we should no longer call them 'foods') and away from traditional, fresh, *real* foods. Therefore, do not let anyone make you feel guilty or shameful about having Type 2 diabetes. You, like millions of others around the world, are a casualty of the distorted food environment in which we now live. As my colleague Dr David Unwin puts it: 'We have eaten our way into this epidemic of diabetes.' We all need support to change what we eat, in order to help us eat our way out of it again.

You may have tried to change your diet several times in the past, and feel that making changes is much easier said than done. I encourage you not to think of needing to 'go on a diet', but of 'making long-term changes to your eating habits that will benefit your health'. The next few chapters will discuss the changes that are most likely to help, but the great news is that you get to choose the detail – which changes you will make and when – to make the change sustainable for you. Your diabetes has probably developed over many years, just as your eating habits have formed over many years, perhaps decades. So, while some people can make massive changes at once, most of us find it easier to make small, manageable changes that, over time, will help us to eat our way out of the ill health associated with diabetes.

Chapter 2

What are the implications of a diagnosis of Type 2 diabetes?

The immediate implications

Uncontrolled Type 2 diabetes is often associated with symptoms such as thirst, excessive urination and blurred vision, due to high glucose levels in the blood. Earlier stages of Type 2 diabetes and prediabetes can be associated with several other, less marked symptoms that may have crept up gradually over years. Even though they are less obvious, they may still have a significant impact on overall wellbeing and health.

One of the most common symptoms that people describe is an overall feeling of lethargy and lack of energy. Often this is combined with difficulty concentrating and thinking clearly. People often assume this is a natural effect of getting older. However, one of the biggest effects reported by people who manage to get their glucose levels down again is that they have much more energy and they can think much more clearly. Poor sleep is also common in people with diabetes, and this can contribute to tiredness and poor concentration. People with high blood glucose levels will often have their sleep disturbed by having to get up to pee several times each night. Apart from the effects of poor sleep, concentration can be affected by a number of factors related to diabetes that affect brain function. It has been shown that mild cognitive impairment is more common in people with raised glucose levels, insulin resistance, obesity and unhealthy eating patterns. A common manifestation of cognitive impairment is 'brain fog', where people find it difficult to concentrate or remember things.

With poor energy levels and poor concentration, it is perhaps not surprising that people with Type 2 diabetes also experience low mood. It is well established that there is a two-way link between depression and Type 2 diabetes, and it has been demonstrated that depressive mood symptoms are worse when blood glucose levels are higher. There is also some evidence that changes in the brains of people with depression can increase the risk of developing Type 2 diabetes, and that clinical depression is at least twice as common in people with diabetes than without.

People whose blood glucose reaches high levels can experience symptoms directly as a result of the effect of high glucose on nerve function. Nerve cells are particularly sensitive to changes in glucose levels, and this can cause tingling, typically in the feet, that can become quite painful. Men can experience erectile dysfunction: high glucose affects the nerves that open up the blood spaces in the penis to cause an erection. These symptoms generally resolve as the blood glucose level improves.

Another effect of a high glucose level is an increased risk and severity of infection. This is particularly common with bladder or genital infections. People with diabetes can also find that skin wounds and insect bites take longer to heal and are more likely to become infected than in people without diabetes.

For most people, the higher infection risk was a nuisance they could live with; all it required was an occasional course of antibiotics. That all changed with the Covid pandemic in 2020. Within a few weeks of the first wave, it became clear that people with diabetes were nearly twice as likely to die of coronavirus than those without diabetes.

Covid highlighted that having Type 2 diabetes has significant effects on the immune system, which weakened its ability to fight the infection. This effect was greatest in people with higher blood glucose levels and who were overweight.

Research has identified that high glucose levels and insulin resistance increase the replication of the Covid virus, reduce the effectiveness of the immune system in targeting the virus, and increase inflammation, causing damage to different organs of the body.

We have known for a long time that people with diabetes have an impaired immune system which puts them at increased risk from infections. However, Covid highlighted that this increased risk is not just a nuisance; it is a potentially deadly effect of having Type 2 diabetes. That is the bad news. The good news is that the two biggest risk factors – having high glucose levels and being overweight – can both be addressed.

The long-term implications

The most important long-term implication of Type 2 diabetes is the development of complications. These are pretty much inevitable in someone whose glucose levels are very high over many years. On the other hand, they can be largely or completely prevented in someone who is able to maintain near-normal levels of blood glucose. In this section, we will briefly discuss the common long-term implications of having Type 2 diabetes. My aim is to provide an accurate account about these complications and their treatment, as well as reassurance that they can be prevented.

The term 'complications of diabetes' refers to the lasting effects of diabetes on various parts of the body. At their worst, they can lead to blindness, kidney failure and amputations. We have known for many years that serious complications are by no means inevitable – especially for someone who is newly diagnosed. In fact, with good management, more severe complications can be avoided altogether, and milder ones can be treated or controlled, ensuring they do not cause any problems. This is because the risk of complications is directly related to the level of glucose in the bloodstream (this is usually assessed by the HbA1c blood test). The higher the HbA1c, the greater the risk. Keeping glucose levels as normal as possible (equivalent to an HbA1c below 50 mmol/mol (or 6.7 per cent)) greatly minimises the risk of complications.

The most important factor in effective management of Type 2 diabetes is lifestyle change from the time of diagnosis: research shows that gains made in this initial phase can have long-lasting health benefits.

Many diabetes-related complications result from vascular disease, which affects the large blood vessels. Atherosclerosis, or narrowing of the arteries, can lead to critical blockages, causing heart attacks or strokes. Lifestyle changes to maintain a normal body weight and stopping smoking can reduce the risk of vascular disease.

Damage to small blood vessels (capillaries) leads to diabetic eye disease (retinopathy), which is the most common complication of diabetes. High glucose levels affect the small blood vessels in the retina at the back of the eyes. In the early stages, vision is not affected, and so regular screening through retinal imaging is essential. In the UK, screening is often provided by high-street optometrists or by mobile units that run screening sessions at different locations. It is free of charge. In other countries, screening is done by eye specialists. Screening enables treatment to be given, if necessary, to prevent retinopathy progressing to cause vision problems.

Diabetic kidney disease (nephropathy) is caused by damage to small blood vessels in the kidneys, impairing their ability to filter waste. Urine tests can detect early signs of protein leaking into urine, indicating kidney damage. Maintaining near-normal levels of glucose and blood pressure, along with medications such as ACE and SGLT2 inhibitors (see Chapter 5), can prevent severe kidney disease and its complications.

Diabetic neuropathy (nerve disease) is caused by high glucose levels damaging nerves, leading to numbness or chronic pain. A simple foot examination to detect loss of sensation is part of routine diabetes care. It is essential that anyone with impaired sensation in their feet examines their feet regularly: they may not feel if they have stepped on a pin, for example, causing a wound that could become infected. Since nerves supply every part of the body, many different body functions can be affected by diabetic nerve damage. One of the most common is for sexual function to be impaired in both men and women. Neuropathy can affect the sweat glands, causing excessive sweating; the bladder, causing frequent urination or difficulty in passing water; and the gut, causing problems such as heartburn, diarrhoea or constipation. Treatments are available that can help control the symptoms of these problems, but they rarely abolish them completely.

Discussing the long-term complications of diabetes is not easy, as they are not very pleasant. However, I believe it is essential that everyone with diabetes knows about them, as appropriate lifestyle changes early on can help people to achieve stable glucose levels – and that is the key to preventing complications from occurring in the first place. It is also essential that people with diabetes go for the regular check-ups that are designed to detect the earliest signs of any of these problems, so they can be addressed before they cause lasting harm.

What can you do to manage Type 2 diabetes?

In short – a huge amount. If you have Type 2 diabetes, this means your body has been struggling to deal with the effects of your lifestyle on your metabolism and your internal organs, as discussed earlier in this section. Doctors used to believe that once you had Type 2 diabetes, it would simply get worse over time, and require more and more medications to keep it under control. But groundbreaking research by Professor Roy Taylor in Newcastle, UK, has shown that this is not the case. He and his team demonstrated that the metabolic and physical changes that lead to Type 2 diabetes can be reversed – and that has huge positive implications on the future health of anyone diagnosed with Type 2 diabetes.

There are many different types of medication that can help reduce glucose levels. While these can make a big difference, they are unlikely to lead to lasting improvements in health unless you make lifestyle changes to allow your body to recover from the effects of your previous way of living. First and foremost, this requires changes to what you eat and drink. The next section will cover the most effective changes, but the most important thing is to reduce your consumption of sugar as much as possible.

Managing diabetes means achieving as near-normal levels of glucose in your blood as possible. This is usually assessed by the HbA1c blood test, which provides an overview of glucose levels over the past two to three months. The UK National Institute of Healthcare and Clinical Excellence (NICE) recommends that management of Type 2 diabetes should aim for an HbA1c between 48 and 53 mmol/mol (6.5 to 7 per cent).

Anyone achieving this level with a combination of medication and lifestyle changes can expect to remain healthy and free from diabetes complications for many years. This in itself is a very exciting prospect for someone who has just been diagnosed with Type 2 diabetes. Even more exciting is the prospect of being able to reverse Type 2 diabetes completely to achieve remission. That means keeping glucose levels below the diabetes range, without the need for medication. The definition of remission is 'achieving and maintaining an HbA1c of less than 48 mmol/mol or 6.5 per cent without the need for any diabetes medication for at least three months'. If that is your goal, the recommendations in this book will help you achieve it. More detailed advice on achieving remission can be found in my book *How to Reverse Type 2 Diabetes and Prediabetes* (see the Appendix). I was recently delighted to hear from a lady who achieved remission in 2014 after reading my first book, *Reverse your Diabetes*. She is still in remission ten years later!

The evidence suggests that the greatest chance of remission is in the first year after diagnosis of Type 2 diabetes. However, it is never too late to make changes to reverse the diabetes disease process to achieve stable and well-managed diabetes (with the help of medication) or to achieve remission (without medication). This includes people who have achieved remission after many years of having diabetes, including some who had been on insulin injections. If you are in that position, you might not be able to achieve full remission, but you have every chance of reversing the process to some extent, resulting in you losing weight, reducing the medication you take, and feeling much better. One of the great results of my approach is that it doesn't just help people to achieve much better control of their diabetes – it also means that many people are able to stop taking medication for other conditions, such as high blood pressure, gout, heartburn or nerve pain in their feet. One person told me, 'My feet feel normal for the first time in years.' And a number of men were delighted to realise that they could perform in the bedroom without the need for Viagra!

Section 2:

A new lifestyle to manage glucose levels

Chapter 3

Diet principles

What is the best diet for Type 2 diabetes?

In Chapter 2, I explained that making changes to your diet is an essential part of managing Type 2 diabetes. However, today so many types of diet are suggested for people with diabetes that it is easy to feel overwhelmed, confused and frustrated. For many years the message from diabetes dietitians and doctors has been that there is no such thing as a 'diabetic diet', and that everyone should 'eat healthily'. That generally means following the advice given to the general population as set out in the National Health Service's Eatwell Guide – essentially a low-fat, high-fibre diet, with around a third of each meal based on starchy carbohydrates.

That is the message that has been given to anyone diagnosed with diabetes in the last thirty years. Anyone diagnosed before then would have been advised to do something very different: to restrict carbohydrates, as it was (and still is) recognised that carbohydrates increase glucose levels in the blood. To switch to advising people with diabetes that all their meals should be based on starchy carbohydrates, when their bodies cannot handle carbohydrates properly, seems very strange. You would think that such a big change in advice would be backed up by high-quality research. I have searched for that research, but in vain. The blunt reality is, it does not exist. I have long believed that this change is a tragic mistake that has led to many people suffering unnecessarily from poor health. And so about fifteen years ago I changed the advice I gave to my own patients. I suggested that they restrict carbohydrates – and they (and I) have never looked back.

Increasingly, more and more doctors and other health professionals now recommend that patients with diabetes restrict the carbs they eat. However, many are still promoting a diet based on the Eatwell Guide, so if you have diabetes, it's easy to become confused about which approach to follow.

Let me explain why I think the advice in the Eatwell Guide (Figure 3.1) is not appropriate for a person with prediabetes or Type 2 diabetes.

Figure 3.1. The Eatwell Guide: official dietary advice from the UK government.

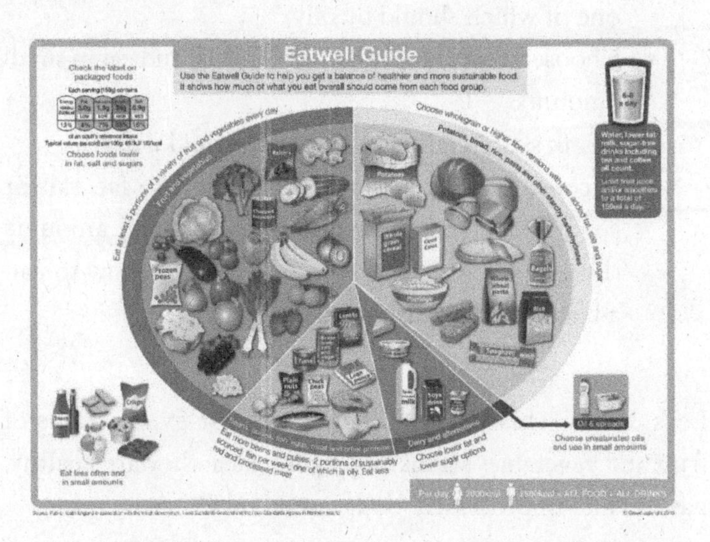

Source: OHID in association with the Welsh government, Food Standards Scotland and the Food Standards Agency in Northern Ireland. Crown copyright.

Its main recommendations are:

- Eat at least five portions of a variety of fruit and vegetables every day.
- Base meals on potatoes, bread, rice, pasta or other starchy carbohydrates, choosing wholegrain versions where possible.
- Have some dairy or dairy alternatives (such as soya drinks), choosing lower fat and lower sugar options.

- Eat some beans, pulses, fish, eggs, meat and other proteins (including two portions of fish every week, one of which should be oily).
- Choose unsaturated oils and spreads, and eat in small amounts.
- Drink six to eight cups/glasses of fluid a day.
- If consuming foods and drinks high in fat, salt or sugar, have these less often and in small amounts (https://www.nhs.uk/live-well/eat-well/how-to-eat-a-balanced-diet/eating-a-balanced-diet/).

Let's discuss these in turn. Eating at least five portions of fruit and vegetables seems like a good idea: they are healthy, natural and unprocessed foods, aren't they?

For leafy and salad vegetables, the answer is yes. Cabbage, courgette (zucchini), cucumber, tomatoes and cauliflower, for example, all have around 3 per cent or less carbohydrate (excluding fibre which, strictly speaking, is a carbohydrate, but is not digested so is not counted). Lettuce, spinach, asparagus, olives and avocado contain even less. Root vegetables such as celeriac or carrots are pretty low at 7 per cent, whereas potatoes are about 15 per cent. But what about fruit? Bananas can be as much as 20 per cent carbs, and grapes are 16 per cent. And raisins are about 75 per cent carbohydrate! Yet in the Eatwell Guide, these are all lumped together.

Why? Because this advice was not designed with its impact on blood glucose levels in mind. According to the Eatwell Guide, fruit and vegetables are all healthy because they contain fibre and plenty of vitamins and minerals. But a tomato or a few chunks of cucumber will have negligible effect on blood glucose levels, whereas a banana could have a massive impact. A large banana could contain up to 40 grams of carbohydrate, yet many people with diabetes have been recommended this as a healthy snack.

Turning to starches, remember these are simply sugar molecules joined together. As soon as they enter your mouth, they begin to break down into glucose. So every one of these foods will increase blood glucose levels. Some, such as bread and white rice, will cause a very rapid rise, while others, such as pasta, will cause a slower one. Even porridge, which is almost universally believed to be a good thing, is over 60 per cent carbohydrate and will cause a big, sustained rise in blood glucose.

The NHS advice is to choose wholegrain versions wherever possible. This is because wholegrains contain more fibre, and this slows down the rise in blood glucose. Yet wholegrain bread and cereals contain so much carbohydrate that they still have a big impact on people with diabetes.

These two categories of food cover three-quarters of the plate. Anyone following the Eatwell Guide will therefore have a high intake of starches – and, depending on the fruit they choose, sugars. What would this type of diet do to the vicious cycle that is the diabetes disease process? Sugars and starches cause blood glucose to rise, prompting the pancreas to release more insulin. High levels of glucose lead to high levels of insulin. High levels of insulin lead to excess energy being stored as fat in the liver. Fat in the liver is a key step in the development of prediabetes and Type 2 diabetes. And so it seems that basing all meals on starchy carbohydrates will only continue that cycle.

It comes as no surprise to me that rates of obesity and Type 2 diabetes have skyrocketed since the 1980s, when dietary guidelines first recommended a low-fat, high-carbohydrate diet. And it doesn't take a genius to work out that eating foods that do not increase blood glucose would be a good change to make. And so, rather than basing all meals on starchy carbohydrates, I firmly believe that the best eating pattern for a person with Type 2 diabetes is one that restricts carbohydrates to a greater or lesser extent, according to personal preference and an individual's goals for their health.

Perhaps because so many people have found that the *official advice* doesn't work, in recent years there has been an explosion in interest in alternative diets. These include plant-based diets, ketogenic (keto) diets (which are very low in carbohydrate and high in fat), low-carbohydrate diets and most recently a carnivore diet (one that excludes all plant-based foods).

Let's discuss this. Since all plant sources of protein (such as beans or lentils) contain carbohydrates, plant-based diets generally involve a higher carbohydrate intake. However, if you reduce or exclude sugars and other refined carbohydrates (such as white bread, pasta and rice) and ultra-processed foods (UPFs), it is perfectly possible to make real health improvements by eating a plant-based diet. However, excluding meat can increase the risk of nutritional deficiencies, such as vitamin B12 or iron, so I generally recommend that people do not exclude meat from their diet – and if they do, to ensure they take any necessary supplements. The other diets (low-carbohydrate, keto and carnivore) are all variations of a low-carbohydrate diet, and different approaches will suit different people.

Healthy choices and how to integrate them

Rather than get bogged down in definitions or precise diet plans, my approach is to suggest a simple, step-by-step approach. Nearly all foods have some effect on blood glucose levels, but by far the biggest culprits are sugars and starches. Therefore, my first recommendation is to reduce these. Since we don't always know what is in processed foods, my second recommendation is to make sure you know what you are eating – and that means eating fresh, unprocessed foods, as far as possible. So, what does that mean in practice?

Cut out sugars

This is essential. If you were one of my patients, one of my first questions would be: are you willing to try to cut out sugars as much as possible? That doesn't mean never eating any foods containing sugar – frankly, that is impossible. But it does mean not including sugary foods as part of your daily diet. Minimising sugars is essential for the good management of prediabetes and Type 2 diabetes.

As we've discussed, diabetes means being intolerant to glucose. If you have coeliac disease, or gluten intolerance, you cannot eat foods that contain gluten. That means avoiding any foods that contain wheat products, including flour. It also means avoiding beer. If you have lactose intolerance, you are advised to avoid all products that contain lactose (milk sugar). By the same token, if you have Type 2 diabetes, you cannot eat sugar. Your body cannot handle it properly. If you have a peanut allergy, you must avoid peanuts *all the time*, otherwise you risk having a massive allergic reaction, which could lead to your death. Diabetes does not act so suddenly. However, eating sugar on a regular basis will increase your blood glucose level and over time will increase your risk of complications – and that carries an increased risk of death. I therefore recommend that you aim to cut out all foods that have added sugars. Apart from the obvious (sugary drinks, sweets, desserts, cakes and biscuits), that also includes many processed foods (such as baked beans). It also includes natural sugars or syrups (such as honey) and fruit that is high in sugar (such as bananas, grapes (unless you can limit yourself to just a few), pineapple and large apples, pears and oranges (small ones are okay, but not ideal). If you are alarmed by the idea of never eating sweet treats again, then you could look into low-sugar alternatives that use artificial sweeteners. Otherwise, save sweet treats for very occasional special occasions. Allow yourself a small piece of cake to celebrate a birthday, and accept that it will cause your glucose level to rise, but that you are willing to take this risk to share in the moment of celebration.

If you have been told that you can eat anything in moderation, and especially if you have been encouraged to eat a lot of fruit, cutting out sugar could mean a big change to your current eating pattern. However, you don't have to change everything in one go. What is important is that you set yourself goals to make changes that are realistic for you, and that you can stick to.

Avoid processed foods

Many processed foods contain high levels of sugars, harmful trans fats, and all sorts of other chemicals. In fact, I have recently heard UPFs being referred to as 'recreational drugs'. Given the lengths to which the food industry goes to make UPFs as tasty and as moreish as possible, this is quite an apt description. I strongly recommend that you try to limit UPFs as much as you can. A good start is to buy foods that do not have an ingredients list (such as fresh meat and vegetables), or to buy foods that have no more than five ingredients (minimally processed foods such as cooked meat, butter or cheese). Butter has just one ingredient – milk – whereas margarine can have twelve or more, including colouring, flavourings, stabilisers and emulsifiers to recreate the buttery taste and texture.

Reduce starches

Starches are found in white or beige foods, including bread, potatoes, rice, pasta, cereals, and any foods that contain flour. Remember that starch is simply glucose molecules stuck together. Some starchy foods, such as white rice, can push up your blood glucose level faster than eating a bowlful of sugar. So, think of a bowl of rice, pasta, breakfast cereal or potatoes as a bowl of sugar: as far as your body is concerned, that is essentially what it is. I recommend that you avoid large portions of starchy foods. This means not eating pasta, rice, pastry, potato-based dishes or large amounts of breakfast cereals. Rather, base your meals on meat or another form of protein and plenty of vegetables, with – at most – a small portion of starchy food as part of the meal. Or experiment with alternatives, such as making 'rice' from grated cauliflower or mixed vegetables with a curry, or courgette strips or leek ribbons instead of pasta.

While white and beige foods contain the highest amounts of starch, smaller amounts are also found in pulses (peas, beans and lentils) and root vegetables (parsnips and carrots). These are high in fibre, which helps reduce their impact on blood glucose levels.

Eat more protein

If you reduce starches in your meals but make no other changes to your diet, then you may find that you go hungry. This is counterproductive, as when you are hungry you could end up eating any food you have available, and that could be high in carbohydrate. So, if you are reducing carbohydrates, make sure you fill up with foods that will not increase the level of glucose in your blood. I usually suggest increasing the portion of protein in your meals. Protein is found in meat, fish, eggs, cheese, pulses and nuts. While protein has some effect in increasing blood glucose levels, it is much less than carbohydrates, so there is no insulin surge to make you hungry again a short time later. Meals that contain protein stay in the stomach for longer so you feel fuller for longer after eating them, and feel less need to snack a couple of hours later. If you do get hungry between meals, try eating a hard-boiled egg or a tinned sardine. They are both inexpensive, nutritious, high-protein, real foods with next to no carbohydrate, and they are very filling – so much so, it is almost impossible to eat a second one. Now, you can't say that about biscuits . . .

Reintroduce fat into your diet

Low-fat foods were introduced in the 1970s, as it was thought that eating saturated fat increased the risk of heart disease. This was called the diet–heart hypothesis, and it led to governments in many countries recommending that we should all eat a low-fat diet. The food industry responded by removing fat from many natural foods, such as dairy products, and adding sugar to make up for their lack of taste – essentially creating a huge array of processed foods. However, more recent studies have questioned the link between fat and heart disease. In 2017, a large study* looked at the diets of over 130,000 people in 18 countries and found that there was no association between fat intake and cardiovascular disease. In fact, a higher fat intake was associated with a reduced risk of death, whereas those who had a higher carbohydrate intake were more likely to die.

---

* Dehghan M, et al. 'Associations of fats and carbohydrate intake with cardiovascular disease and mortality in 18 countries from five continents (PURE): a prospective cohort study.' *Lancet*, 2017, 390(10107): 2050–62.

Many people believe that fat is bad. I have had to repeat to many of my patients that it is not just okay to eat fat, but it's better than eating carbohydrates. There are many different types of fat – monounsaturated, polyunsaturated (omega 3 and omega 6), saturated and trans fats. While some are definitely bad, most are now recognised to be very good for us.

Monounsaturated fat is found in olives, seeds and various types of nut. Nuts have a low carbohydrate content, and are quite high in (mainly healthy) fats, meaning they satisfy the appetite: a handful of nuts is a good snack. The Mediterranean diet is rich in monounsaturated fats and has several health benefits. A major study published in 2013 demonstrated that eating a Mediterranean diet was associated with a 30 per cent reduction in cardiovascular events (e.g. heart attacks or strokes) compared to eating a low-fat diet.* What is also overlooked or understated is that about half of the fat in meat is also monounsaturated.

Polyunsaturated fat comes in two types. One type is omega 3, which is healthy fat and may help lower the risk of heart disease, depression, dementia and arthritis. Your body can't make it, so you must eat foods that contain it. It is found in oily fish, and ideally should be eaten two to three times a

* Estruch R, Ros E, Salas-Salvado J, et al. 'Primary prevention of cardiovascular disease with a Mediterranean diet.' *N. Engl. J. Med.*, 2013, 368: 1279–90.

week. Nuts (especially walnuts) and linseed (flaxseed) are also a good source of omega 3. The other type of polyunsaturated fat is omega 6, which is less beneficial. It is found in vegetable oils and spreads containing corn oil or sunflower oil. Eating too many foods containing omega 6 fats can increase inflammation in the body.

Saturated fat is found in dairy products and meat, as well as coconut and, in small amounts, even in avocado. Recent research has shown that saturated fat is not the enemy we once thought it was: it is not associated with an increased risk of heart disease.* It also increases healthy high-density lipoprotein (HDL) cholesterol levels. In natural foods such as unprocessed meat, it can be considered a healthy fat.

Trans fats (also known as hydrogenated fats) are the real baddies. Although they occur in small quantities in some natural foods, such as meat and dairy products, man-made versions are found in many processed foods. They have been shown to increase inflammation and the risk of heart disease. A number of food manufacturers are reducing their use of trans fats, but they can still be found in many baked products and margarines and in foods fried in vegetable oils.

---

* de Souza RJ, Mente A, Maroleanu A, et al. 'Intake of saturated and trans unsaturated fatty acids and risk of all cause mortality, cardiovascular disease, and type 2 diabetes: systematic review and meta-analysis of observational studies.' *BMJ*, 2015, 351: h3978.

Adding healthy fats to your diet can help to make meals more filling. Naturally occurring fats as found in oily fish, nuts, avocado and olives are considered healthy. Adding some of these can make a salad into a delicious, filling meal. Fat also has virtually no effect on blood glucose or insulin levels.

So what about cheese? There is now evidence from a number of studies* that dairy products are not harmful to our health, and some, such as yoghurt and cheese, may actually be associated with a lower risk of heart disease. Therefore, you can eat cheese. I have lost count of the number of people who express surprise or shock when I say to them, 'Why not eat some cheese?' They feel liberated after many years of being told not to eat cheese, or of only eating low-fat cheeses. I would much rather my patients have a small piece of cheese as a snack than a sweet biscuit. Of course, if you eat a lot of cheese, or other dairy products, then you will gain weight. Since cheese (like nuts) contains small amounts of carbohydrate, it can be rather moreish, and if you are not careful you can end up eating quite a lot. But a small piece of cheese, preferably without a cracker, is a delicious and healthy way to round off a meal.

---

* Forouhi NG, Krauss RM, Taubes G, Willett W. 'Dietary fat and cardiometabolic health: evidence, controversies, and consensus for guidance.' *BMJ*, 2018, 361: k2139.

In summary, dairy products, nuts, seeds, oily fish and meat all contain healthy natural fats and can be enjoyed as part of your eating plan.

Don't count calories

Most weight-loss diets are based on the principle that you take in fewer calories in food and drink and you use up more calories by physical activity than you eat, so you lose weight. Many diets encourage you to count the calories in the foods you eat, to ensure you stick to a certain number. In my experience, many people find such diets hard to follow, and they often do not work.

These diets assume that a calorie from fat has the same effect on your body as a calorie from protein or carbohydrate. For a person with diabetes, this is a huge oversimplification. We have already heard that protein and fat have a much smaller effect on glucose levels than carbohydrate, and so the body will release much more insulin after a small portion of rice that contains 200 calories than after a piece of cheese that also contains 200 calories. Remember, insulin is the fat storage hormone, and so more fat is likely to be stored after eating 200 calories in rice than in cheese. Insulin also promotes hunger, so you are more likely to want to eat more after eating rice. A few years ago Sam Feltham, Director of the UK's Public Health Collaboration, did a single-person experiment to assess how different types of foods affect weight. He ate 5,800 calories a day for twenty-one days on different diets. When he ate a low-carb, high-fat diet his weight increased by 1.3 kg, yet when he ate a low-fat, high-carbohydrate diet, his weight increased by 7.1 kg! But the number of calories he ate was the same. He noted that on the low-carbohydrate diet he wasn't hungry and often had to force himself to eat to make up his target calorie count.

This demonstrates how, through the action of insulin, carbohydrates have a bigger impact on hunger and on body weight than other nutrients. And yet most calorie-controlled diets completely ignore the role of insulin.

In addition, some foods use up more energy in their digestion than others. Protein requires up to 30 per cent of its calories to digest it, whereas carbohydrate requires about 10 per cent. So, if you have 200 calories as protein – as in a 200-gram (7-ounce) steak, for example – 60 of those calories are burned off in the digestion process, meaning your body only gets to use 140 of them. On the other hand, only 10 per cent of calories are burned off digesting carbohydrate (20 calories in a small portion of rice). These flaws in the low-calorie argument have led many of us to believe that a calorie in rice or sugar is much more harmful than a calorie in steak or cream – or, put another way, not all calories are the same in how they affect your weight.

If you significantly reduce your calorie intake, say to 800 calories a day, then you will lose weight. But many people find that they can also lose a lot of weight simply by reducing the carbohydrates in their diet. Replacing starchy carbs with green vegetables is a great start and will reduce your insulin level, which is key to losing weight, because it reverses the vicious cycle of the diabetes disease process.

So, I suggest that you don't need to count calories. Reducing carbs will likely also reduce the calories you eat. Having said that, it is important to be aware of which low-carbohydrate foods are high in calories, such as cheese or nuts, and to limit your intake of these if you are finding it difficult to lose weight.

Making a start with your new diet

So, cutting out sugars and avoiding large portions of starches is essential for the effective management of Type 2 diabetes. But how you set about doing that is entirely up to you. Some people choose to cut out all starchy foods and eat a very low-carbohydrate, ketogenic diet. Others follow a carnivore diet – eating only meat, eggs and dairy products. Both will lead to an immediate and dramatic reduction in glucose levels, but some people can find these diets too restrictive, and the evidence suggests they are unnecessary for many people. Making severe reductions to carbohydrate intake can lead to some side effects, such as constipation, muscle cramps and headaches. These usually subside after a few days and can be eased by drinking plenty of fluids.

So, rather than reducing carbohydrates as much as possible, the most important thing is to choose an eating plan that you think you will be able to stick to over the long term. It is perfectly possible to manage, and in many cases reverse, Type 2 diabetes while still enjoying small amounts of starch in your diet. Many people prefer to make gradual changes to their diet. I have developed a step-by-step approach to reducing carbohydrates. This approach addresses the most important changes first. However, it is not the only way. You may feel that Step 4 is the easiest change for you to make – if so, start with Step 4 rather than Step 1.

Please note that if you take any medications for diabetes, it is essential that you read Chapter 5 before you make any changes to your diet.

Step 1: Stop drinking sugary drinks

Cutting out added sugars is probably the most important first step to stabilising your glucose levels. If you drink sugary drinks, these should be the first thing to stop. There is enough scientific evidence that sugar-sweetened beverages are harmful that I recommend to my patients that they cut them out completely. In addition to the obvious examples, such as Coke and other types of fizzy drink, this also means cutting out fruit juices and smoothies – despite the health benefits they may have. We have already discussed how some fruits are not a healthy option if you have diabetes, but any fruit, when turned into a smoothie, becomes a very sweet drink, albeit with some fibre in it. In terms of sugar content, smoothies are on a par with Coke. It does not matter that the sugar is 'natural' (that is, it originally came from fruit) – it is still sugar, and will have a big impact on the level of glucose, and therefore insulin, in your bloodstream. This also means cutting out sweetened hot drinks, such as hot chocolate, lattes and flavoured cappuccinos available in popular coffee shops.

There are not many things that I suggest avoiding completely, but sweet drinks are one of them. I would even say that I don't think it's possible to manage Type 2 diabetes if you continue to drink sugar in this way. If you like sugary drinks, please consider switching to diet versions that use artificial sweeteners as a first step in reducing your sugar intake. Sweeteners can also cause problems, but they are a much better option than sugar.

To minimise liquid sugar intake, the best drinks are water or unsweetened tea (including fruit or herbal teas) or coffee with a dash of milk. To add flavour to a glass of water, try adding a slice of lemon, lime or cucumber.

Step 2: Reduce snacking

The next stage is to cut right down on sugar. Many natural foods have small amounts of sugar, so it is not possible to avoid sugar completely. However, you can try to avoid foods with added sugar, such as sweets, biscuits, cakes, ice cream and desserts, as well as sweet fruit. A lot of these foods are snacks rather than main meals so, rather than focusing on a long list of foods that you need to avoid, I encourage you to think of it another way: as cutting out snacks.

Snacks were invented by the food industry to maximise their profits by getting us to eat food we don't need, and they throw hundreds of millions of pounds annually at developing and marketing them. As a child, I remember being told not to snack as it would 'spoil my appetite'; now we are encouraged to get through tons of snacks, many of which are ultra-processed and high in sugar. As a relatively recent grandad, I have noticed that toddlers cannot go anywhere without an ultra-processed (and often marketed as 'organic') snack readily available, and so we are teaching future generations that this is normal. It is not.

Instead, I encourage you to focus on eating enough at your main meals to fill you up, thus avoiding the need for any food between meals. That means having your mid-morning cup of tea or coffee on its own, without a biscuit, banana or bar of chocolate, or, if you are in a coffee shop, a cake or pastry. Remember, we do not *need* any of these foods: we eat them because we like them, and quite often because it has become a habit. Yes, we might enjoy the taste and the sugar rush that comes with the first few mouthfuls, but then we might feel rather bloated and uncomfortable afterwards. Try having a drink without a snack – you will find that you can still enjoy your drink, and as it fills your stomach it will make you feel full, but without feeling as if you have overdone it.

If you eat biscuits, chocolate or cake between meals, then cutting them out will reduce your sugar intake very significantly. This will reduce your blood glucose level, which in turn will reduce your insulin level. This means you will feel less hungry between meals, with less need to snack. This means your glucose level will stay down and you will likely lose weight. Win–win!

There will be times when you feel peckish, so it's important to ensure you have some healthier snacks available. Examples include a small piece of cheese, a few strawberries, some vegetable sticks, a handful of nuts, a hard-boiled egg or a piece of dark chocolate.

Maybe you do not eat cakes or biscuits, but you enjoy eating fruit – perhaps five or more pieces a day. You may be thinking you are doing the right thing, as all the official advice is to eat fruit. However, some fruit – such as banana, pineapple and mango – are very high in sugar and are best avoided, unless you can restrict yourself to a very small portion. A single grape is low in carbohydrate, and as long as you eat no more than five at a time, this should be fine: however, if stopping at five is difficult, then it's best to avoid grapes. Instead, get your five a day from vegetables rather than fruit. If you want to reduce your sugar levels, remember: berries are best, as they are very low in sugar, followed by small apples, plums or tangerines – or any fruit that you can easily fit in the palm of your hand. Dried fruit (such as prunes, raisins and dried apricots), on the other hand, is very high in sugar, so it is best avoided.

Whether you have a sugar addiction, have a sweet tooth, or simply enjoy eating sweet treats, you might find it difficult to cut out all sugary foods completely. If that is the case, then start by identifying one or two small changes that you think you can make. It could be having one instead of two biscuits or having an apple instead of a pastry. It doesn't matter what the change is, so long as it is one that you think you can achieve. However, if you genuinely feel addicted to certain foods, the aim should be that eventually you stop them completely, however difficult that might seem.

Step 3: Have less starch for breakfast

For many people, reducing their sugar intake will have a big effect in improving their glucose levels, which is great. Many others will have cut out a lot of sugary foods when they developed Type 2 diabetes or prediabetes. However, they may also be consuming a lot of starchy foods – after all, that was probably the advice they received. Remember that starch is simply sugar molecules joined together and, like sugar, it increases the glucose and insulin levels in the blood. Reducing starchy foods is therefore an essential part of managing Type 2 diabetes and reversing the disease process.

For Step 3, I suggest focusing on breakfast to start with. There is a very good reason for this. Whenever I ask people what they eat for breakfast, most say they have starch, in the form of cereal and/or toast. However, breakfast is the worst possible time to challenge the body with carbohydrates. At this time, the levels of many hormones – such as cortisol and growth hormone – are quite high. I call them the 'wake up' hormones as they prepare the body for the day ahead, and part of the way they work is to counter the effect of insulin. That means, if you have Type 2 diabetes or prediabetes, insulin resistance is worse at breakfast time than at any other time of the day.

For many people, 'breakfast' means having a breakfast cereal. That was my standard breakfast for countless years. But if you stop to look at the ingredients you will see they are all processed foods. Many so-called 'healthy' options, such as muesli, contain dried fruit and are very high in sugar (even when labelled 'no added sugar'), and they are all very high in starch. As far as your body is concerned, you might as well be eating a bowlful of sugar. After cereal we might also eat toast, each slice being 15–20 grams of carbohydrate. So a breakfast of a bowl of cereal and couple of slices of toast easily adds up to 80 or 90 grams of carbohydrate, in just one meal, at a time of day when your body is least able to deal with it.

The most important advice I can give here is to stop eating breakfast cereals – all of them, including the 'healthy' ones, and even porridge. Plain (full-fat) Greek yoghurt with some mixed berries is a natural, filling, healthier alternative, with a fraction of the carbohydrate content. If you have time to cook, bacon and eggs or a mushroom omelette will fill you up with practically zero carbs! Another zero-carb option, of course, is to skip breakfast, if you prefer a time-restricted eating regime (as we will discuss in Chapter 6). Despite what you may have been told, missing breakfast can be good for you. Are you willing to give it a try, maybe once a week?

Step 4: Have a low-carb lunch

Just as breakfast can add up to a huge carb load, so also can lunch – or what has become a usual lunch for many of us.

A sandwich, packet of crisps and a piece of fruit can easily total over 80 grams of carbohydrate. So what are the options to reduce carbs at lunchtime, especially if you are out and about, when it can be very difficult to buy a low-carb lunch? Some people ask if a wrap is a better option than a sandwich, and the answer is no: a wrap can easily contain the same, if not more, carbohydrate than two slices of bread. The same goes for crackers or crispbread. While they are small and thin, they are basically concentrated flour, and therefore very high in carbohydrate.

If you want a low-carbohydrate lunch, you really need to move away from flour-based foods. My advice is to have soup or salad. A salad has very few carbs, and if you choose carefully, many soups are also low-carb, especially if they are homemade. Homemade soup, especially vegetable soup, is remarkably easy to make – even if you don't consider yourself to be a great cook – and is usually very tasty. You can make up a large quantity and take it to work in a container to microwave, or in an insulated flask. For salads, I generally say: have whatever you would have put in your sandwich, but with some lettuce and tomato instead of bread. Add a hard-boiled egg and you have a high-protein (and therefore very filling) low-carb lunch.

Rather than going to the sandwich aisle for lunch, go to the cooked meat or cheese section. Many supermarkets now sell cooked chicken thighs or drumsticks and slices of ham or cheese that can be eaten 'on the go'. Another option, but one that's less easy to eat on the move, is tinned fish. One of my patients once told me that they take a tin of sardines to work for lunch. It might not be as easy to eat as a sandwich, but with a bit of care, you can eat sardines from the tin at your desk. They are packed with protein and healthy fats, with near-zero carbohydrate. They will likely keep you full right into the evening. In the UK at least, they are also very cheap, at around 60p for a 125 g tin of sardines in olive oil or brine – much cheaper than any shop-bought sandwich or meal deal.

If you can't avoid eating a sandwich for lunch, I suggest eating sandwiches with the most generous fillings, and eat as few as you need to feel satiated. If you can, leave the crusts. Or if you're at home, try some of the lower-carb breads that are now available, or buy one of the low-carb alternatives to flour – these can be used to make very passable bread.

Step 5: Think 'meat and two veg'

When it comes to main meals, my advice is to think of 'meat and two veg' type meals rather than meals based on potatoes, pasta or rice. Perhaps 'protein and as many veg as you can manage' would be a better description. This is designed to include meals for non-meat eaters and to make it clear that you can pile your plate with as many veg as you like. So, any type of meat, poultry, fish, seafood, pulses, nuts, seeds, cheese or eggs prepared in any way you choose, together with an array of fresh or frozen vegetables. The only caveat is: avoid flour-based sauces, and be mindful that root vegetables contain starch. Even so, you can occasionally add a few small new potatoes or chips, if you really can't manage without them. It's as simple as that! The way potatoes are cooked affects their carbohydrate content. Boiled potatoes absorb water, thus reducing their carb content, whereas roasting or frying dehydrates them and makes the carbohydrate more concentrated. So, having a few small roast potatoes could have a much bigger effect on glucose levels than choosing the same number of boiled potatoes.

If you enjoy pasta or rice-based meals, then you can adapt them to use vegetable alternatives (ribbons of leek as a substitute for spaghetti, linguine or tagliatelle, for example). If you love takeaway curries, you can still enjoy many of these dishes, although be aware that some may contain sugar. Instead of having rice with a curry, try curried mixed vegetables or non-starchy sides such as saag bhaji or cauliflower bhaji, or a bed of shredded lettuce. Try to consciously (re) train your mind and stomach to believe that curries don't have to be served with rice or chapattis. Some people make cauliflower 'rice' by stir-frying grated cauliflower. Invest in a spiraliser to make courgette 'spaghetti' to enjoy with your Bolognese sauce instead of pasta. And instead of mashed potato on shepherd's pie, try mashed celeriac or cauliflower – they have only a fraction of the carbohydrate found in potato.

If you wish to reduce your carbohydrate intake to a very low level, then you will need to take into account the carbohydrates found in vegetables. Broadly speaking, leafy and salad vegetables have the lowest carbs, whereas legumes (peas, beans and lentils) and root vegetables contain higher levels.

I suggest that you try to manage without desserts; if you eat a good main meal following the above guidelines, your body won't need a dessert. If you do fancy one, though, then berries with full-fat Greek yoghurt, crème fraiche or double cream are all very tasty, low-carb options. If you are having a special meal, then there are a number of low-carb dessert recipes available. Emma Porter at thelowcarbkitchen.co.uk has a recipe for a delicious chocolate mousse made with coconut milk or whipped cream and 90 per cent dark chocolate. She also has recipes for low-carb crackers if you prefer cheese after a meal. Alternatively, eat cheese with celery instead of crackers.

Step 6: Watch what you drink

We have already discussed the need to reduce sugar in soft drinks and hot drinks. But what about alcohol? If you have Type 2 diabetes or prediabetes, the recommendations around alcohol are the same as for everyone else: to limit your intake to 14 units a week or less. However, it is important to be aware that alcohol is very efficient at filling the liver with fat, which is one of the key steps in the diabetes disease process. Alcohol is also very high in calories. So if you want to lose weight, and especially if you drink in excess of 14 units a week, reducing your intake will certainly help. Some people choose to stop drinking alcohol altogether for a while as part of their journey to improved health.

If you drink alcohol, then it is important to know what effect your drinks will have on your blood glucose levels. Since alcohol is produced by fermentation of sugar, then as a rough rule of thumb, the higher the alcohol content, the lower the sugar content. Therefore, most spirits that are high in alcohol have no sugar in them. Dry red or white wine has a low sugar content and should not adversely affect your glucose levels, especially if drunk with a meal. Beer contains carbohydrate, and so I generally advise beer drinkers to consider beer like any other carb-containing food and avoid drinking large quantities. The highest sugar levels are found in cider, sweet liqueurs, alcopops and some low-alcohol wines and beers – these are best avoided altogether.

Chapter 4

The role of exercise

Many of my patients who are overweight or have high glucose levels tell me that it is because they do not exercise enough. They are often quite surprised when I tell them that exercise is unlikely to help them lose weight or reduce their glucose levels. That requires making the changes to your diet we have discussed.

Exercise is great for your heart and for building muscle strength. It is also great for mental health and wellbeing. But it is not great for losing weight or controlling diabetes. Studies show it has only a small effect. In fact, anaerobic exercise such as weight training or very high-intensity exercise can actually increase blood glucose levels, so can be counterproductive for people with Type 2 diabetes. For people who are very overweight, exercise can pose a real risk of injury.

That is why I do not talk about exercise when I speak to people who want to lose weight or reduce their glucose levels. Too many people have negative connotations around exercise: failure, pain, Lycra, having to go to a gym, embarrassment about body image in the changing room, and so on. People are usually very happy when I say don't exercise. Instead, I recommend they *walk*. Not a brisk walk; just a walk. If a patient is unable to walk, I recommend that they move as much as possible using chair-based exercises. Any physical activity will do.

Back in the 1950s, research showed that people who walked as part of their job were healthier than people who sat down all day. One famous study looked at the health of two groups of workers on London buses: drivers (who spent several hours sitting behind the steering wheel) and conductors, whose job was to sell tickets to passengers, moving along the rows of seats and up and down the stairs all day long. The study also looked at postmen, who spent much of their day walking to deliver mail, and telephone switchboard operators who, like bus drivers, were seated during their working hours. They found that more active workers (postmen and bus conductors) had lower death rates from heart disease than their less active colleagues.*

More recently, the beneficial effects of physical activity on metabolic health were emphasised by a study from Denmark,

* Morris JN, Heady JA, et al. 'Coronary heart disease and physical activity at work.' *Lancet*, 1953, 1053–7.

in which active healthy volunteers were persuaded to reduce their activity from over 10,000 steps a day to less than 1,500. After just two weeks they had higher blood insulin levels and a significant increase in abdominal fat,* both precursors to the development of Type 2 diabetes. So you can see that walking is good for metabolic health.

Walk your way to better health

But sitting down is not. In one study, over 500 adults with newly diagnosed Type 2 diabetes were asked to wear an accelerometer – a wearable device that measures activity levels. They also had various other measurements performed to assess their overall metabolic health. The accelerometers were analysed to determine how long they were inactive. The study concluded that the longer they sat down each day, the higher the level of insulin in their blood and the worse their insulin resistance. This inactive time was also associated with an increase in waist circumference of nearly 2 cm (about 0.75 of an inch) and with a reduction in healthy HDL cholesterol – both known consequences of insulin resistance.† This

---

* Olsen RH, et al. 'Metabolic responses to reduced daily steps in healthy nonexercising men.' *JAMA*, 2008, 299: 1261.

† Healy GN, Dunstan DW, et al. 'Breaks in sedentary time: beneficial associations with metabolic risk.' *Diabetes Care*, 2008, 31(4): 661–6.

suggests that the more time we spend sitting down, the more likely we are to develop Type 2 diabetes. Indeed, this was the conclusion of a meta-analysis of a number of studies that looked at the effect of time spent watching TV on people's health. This showed that, on average, for every two hours spent watching television each day, the risk of developing Type 2 diabetes increased by 20 per cent, and the risk of death from all causes increased by 13 per cent. Incredibly, people who spent five hours a day watching television had a 50 per cent increased risk of developing diabetes.* The same likely applies to people who sit behind a screen all day at work.

Since we now know that the changes that lead to Type 2 diabetes can be reversed, my advice to anyone with Type 2 diabetes is to move more and to sit less.

Walking is the ideal physical activity. It is free, does not require any special equipment, and is, lest we forget, a very useful form of transport. My focus is not on 'going out for a walk' – unless you are predominantly based at home – as that requires you to make the time to fit a walk into your daily routine. Rather, I encourage everyone to build walking into their daily routine. You can do this by:

---

* Grøntved A, Hu FB. 'Television viewing and risk of type 2 diabetes, cardiovascular disease, and all-cause mortality: a meta-analysis.' *JAMA*, 2011, 305(23): 2448–55.

- If you use the bus, tram or Underground (metro or subway), get off at least one stop before you need to, so that you have to walk part of your journey.
- If driving somewhere, find a place to park a few hundred metres from where you need to be.
- If shopping at a supermarket or other store with a large car park, park as far away from the store entrance as you can.
- Choose to walk or cycle rather than use a car for any trips less than 2 km (1.5 miles).
- Use stairs rather than lifts or escalators.

If you are not used to walking, then I recommend that you choose one or two of these changes and give them a try. Remember, you don't have to walk briskly; walking at any speed is better than not walking at all. If you are overweight, then your knees or hips may ache to start with. But as you lose weight, these aches and pains should ease.

You might then try going out for a walk after lunch or your evening meal, as a way to use up the energy from the meal and minimise the rise in blood glucose that otherwise might occur. Even a fifteen-minute walk can help keep your blood glucose level stable after a meal.

The more you walk, the more your strength will improve and the easier and more enjoyable you will find it. Only a short walk significantly increases brain activity and, with it, a feeling of wellbeing. Research has shown that being in green spaces also improves health and wellbeing. That doesn't have to mean a walk in the country; it could be in a town park, or along a river bank or even a tree-lined street, so if you can include these on your walking route, then you will have added benefit.

Sit down less

My first message around physical activity is to walk more. My second is to sit down less – or, specifically, to try to avoid sitting for longer than an hour at a time. So many of us spend several hours each day, whether at work or at home, sitting in front of a screen, whether a television or a computer. Again, this is a huge change from just a few decades ago. Anyone aged over forty will remember a time when most homes did not have a computer, and anyone over thirty will remember a time when a mobile phone pretty much only made phone calls. The advent of laptops, smartphones and the internet mean that for many of us, work, play, shopping and socialising can all be done from the sofa, where we can spend hours on end, sitting, slouching or lying down. This is called sedentary time, and it is bad for our health.

If watching more television increases the risk of Type 2 diabetes, then you would hope that reducing the amount of time you spend watching television would have the opposite effect. Support for this comes from a small study from the United States in which a group of thirty-six overweight people (with a body mass index (BMI) of between 25 and 50), who watched TV on average for three hours each day, were randomly split into a control group and an intervention group. The intervention group were asked to reduce their television viewing time by 50 per cent. After three weeks, this group were found to have significantly increased their energy expenditure (measured using an accelerometer) and to have lost some weight.*

Even if you don't watch television, modern life means that long periods of sedentary time are inevitable for many people – for example, people whose jobs involve driving or sitting at a desk. What can these people do to try to preserve their health? Studies have looked at the effect of 'breaks' in sedentary time. Research has shown that people who interrupted their sedentary time, even for only a minute, reduced their waist circumference, body weight and blood glucose levels, but people who did not interrupt their seated time did

---

* Otten JJ, Jones KE, et al. 'Effects of television viewing reduction on energy intake and expenditure in overweight and obese adults.' *Arch. Intern. Med.*, 2009, 169(22): 2109–15.

not.* There are several possible reasons for this, including the fact that the act of standing, even for a short time, uses significantly more energy than sitting down. I explain this using an analogy with a computer. If you do not use your computer for a certain length of time, it goes into sleep mode. That is, it is still on, but the screen has switched off and the processors have stopped processing and the fans have stopped whirring to *conserve* energy. In the same way, if we do not use our body for a period, our metabolism goes into a sort of sleep mode, and slows down to use only enough energy to keep things ticking over. As a result, blood glucose levels rise and the energy saved is stored as fat in the liver – hence the increased waist circumference. The simple act of standing up has a similar effect to moving your computer's mouse: it wakes up your body, which starts operating again at full speed, consuming more energy as it does.

Take regular breaks if you sit all day

Try to avoid sitting down for longer than an hour. This means that if you are sitting at work all day, at your desk or in a meeting, or in front of the TV at home, remind yourself to stand up at least once an hour and walk around for a

---

* Cooper RS, Sebire S, et al. 'Sedentary time, breaks in sedentary time and metabolic variables in people with newly diagnosed type 2 diabetes.' *Diabetologia*, 2012, 55: 589–99.

couple of minutes, before sitting down again and continuing to do what you were doing. You don't even have to leave the room – although if you do venture outside for a couple of minutes, it will boost your system in other ways as well. Many people set their watch or their phone to buzz every hour to remind them to get up. At work, I suggest that people make their office as *inefficient* as possible, so that the printer or filing cabinet are not right next to their desk. Better still, use a standing desk, or an adjustable height desk so that you can work at it while standing.

Many of my patients are delighted when I say 'don't exercise, don't even think of joining a gym, simply walk more and sit less' – but as they then lose weight, they find they can walk further without any accompanying aches and pains or shortness of breath. They feel healthier and better about themselves and many choose to become more adventurous: they might dig out an old bike to rediscover how much they once enjoyed cycling; or they may join a local community run (such as Parkrun), knowing that it is perfectly okay to walk or to stop/start. No one is judging. Other initiatives include Couch to 5K (C25K): an exercise plan that gradually progresses from beginner running towards a 5-kilometre run over nine weeks. There are also walking football and walking netball, created to enable people to enjoy the games they used to love playing, but at a walking pace.

I mentioned earlier that exercise is good for overall health, and as you lose weight and become more mobile, you may find yourself wanting to begin a regime of more intensive exercise or join a gym or an exercise class. All exercise is good, provided you don't get over-ambitious and risk injuring yourself. Do whatever you find enjoyable! If you enjoy the exercise you do, you are more likely to keep it up.

But to repeat: for weight loss and improved glucose levels I recommend moderate cardio exercise such as walking or jogging. It is important to be aware that more intensive exercise – and anaerobic exercise, such as strength training – can actually increase glucose levels. However, yoga and Pilates have been shown to be beneficial for people with Type 2 diabetes. They incorporate strength training but in a relaxed way, so they help reduce glucose levels.

Perhaps you feel that participating in any kind of exercise is too much to contemplate. And that is absolutely fine. Yet . . . please consider what changes you could make in your day-to-day life to *walk more* and *sit less*. And when you feel motivated to do something more energetic, come back and have another look at this chapter.

Chapter 5

The role of medication

For many years, medication has been the main treatment for people with Type 2 diabetes. Even though most official guidelines recommend changing your diet and being more active, these usually get only a token mention while the rest is all about medication. The UK NICE guidelines for the management of Type 2 diabetes are forty-nine pages long: two pages discuss diet while forty-four pages cover various medications. It is therefore unsurprising that many health professionals consider medication to be the more important approach. From what I have said already, it should be clear that I hold a different view: I firmly believe that the most important part of treating anyone with Type 2 diabetes is dietary change. No medication will work if the person taking it is eating foods that push up their glucose levels. For many people, making changes to their diet is enough to manage Type 2 diabetes very well, and for some, it enables them to achieve remission of diabetes. However, it is important to acknowledge that many people will require medication to enable them to manage their diabetes. For these people, I always emphasise that the role of medication is to help the dietary changes – not the other way round. This is a crucial distinction and is one reason why I encourage people to make changes to their diet when they are first diagnosed with Type 2 diabetes, before starting medication. Some doctors believe that everyone should start metformin tablets at the time of diagnosis. I disagree, since I believe this could lead to a mindset that 'diabetes is treated with tablets', with dietary changes seen as an optional extra.

Bearing this in mind, I will now describe the medications that can help in the management of Type 2 diabetes.

What you will be prescribed

Over the past twenty years, a number of new medications have been developed to treat Type 2 diabetes. As a result, there are now plenty of options that work in different ways. This is very different from the situation when I first started working in diabetes, when there were essentially three treatments: metformin, a group of drugs called sulfonylureas (which make the pancreas produce extra insulin), and insulin. Given our current understanding – that the main problem in Type 2 diabetes is that the body produces too much insulin – it does not make sense to use treatments that increase insulin still further, as this makes it almost impossible for a person using these treatments to reverse the diabetes disease process. In my practice, I prescribe sulfonylureas and insulin much less nowadays.

Metformin

The first of the original trio, metformin, is still very much in use. In fact, although it is one of the oldest diabetes treatments available (it was first used in the 1950s), almost every treatment guideline from around the world recommends it as the first drug to be prescribed for people with Type 2 diabetes. Unlike sulfonylureas, metformin does not increase the amount of insulin the pancreas produces. Rather, it helps the body use its own insulin more effectively, thus reducing insulin resistance. This means the pancreas does not need to produce so much insulin to control blood glucose levels – and less insulin makes it easier to lose weight. Two other types of drug commonly in use today, dipeptidyl peptidase-4 (DPP4) inhibitors and glucagon-like peptide-1 (GLP1) analogues, also work by reducing insulin resistance.

Pioglitazone is another drug that reduces insulin resistance, but as it causes weight gain and other side effects, it is used less often now.

SGLT2 inhibitors

The newest diabetes drugs are known as sodium-glucose co-transporter-2 (SGLT2) inhibitors. They work by making the kidneys remove additional glucose from the bloodstream and pass it into the urine. They therefore reduce blood glucose levels directly, which in turn reduces the amount of insulin that needs to be produced: consequently, they also help with weight loss. Acarbose, which is rarely used nowadays as it can cause unpleasant gut side effects, reduces glucose levels by stopping it from being absorbed from the gut into the bloodstream.

Because of their impact on reducing the level of insulin in the blood, metformin, DPP4 inhibitors, GLP1 analogues and SGLT2 inhibitors can all help reverse the diabetes disease process. The following table lists the most common drugs used in 2024 to treat Type 2 diabetes in the UK. Note that all have side effects. In many people these are relatively mild, such as nausea or abdominal bloating. But some drugs, in certain situations, can have quite serious side effects. For example, SGLT2 inhibitors can be associated with a serious metabolic condition known as diabetic ketoacidosis in people with naturally low insulin levels. It is therefore essential that everyone who takes medication is aware of the potential side effects, so they can make an informed decision about whether that medicine is right for them.

Table 5.1 lists the most commonly used types of diabetes medication. As already mentioned, metformin is the drug of first choice. Metformin is generally started at a low dose – for example, one 500 mg tablet daily – and increased over a few weeks to the maximum dose of 1 gram twice daily. It is inexpensive, and in most people it's effective and safe; however, it is important to be aware of its side effects, which mostly affect the gut. Usually these are mild and limited to bloating, wind and mild diarrhoea. The side effects can be reduced by taking metformin with food and by using slow-release preparations. Side effects generally settle once the gut has got used to the medication, but if they do not, then metformin should be stopped and an alternative drug used instead. Metformin cannot be used by people with significantly reduced kidney function. It does not work immediately, so do not expect an instant improvement in glucose levels: it can take a few weeks for its effects to become apparent.

Once a person is established on metformin, some guidelines recommend that anyone with heart or kidney problems (whether related to diabetes or not) should also start taking an SGLT2 inhibitor. In addition to helping reduce glucose levels, they are effective in reducing blood pressure and protecting the heart and kidneys from further damage. Both metformin and SGLT2 inhibitors must be stopped if you become acutely unwell: for example, with a severe infection, or vomiting or diarrhoea causing dehydration. They can usually be restarted once you have recovered.

For people who are started on metformin alone, an SGLT2 inhibitor can be added if glucose levels remain too high. The decision to add an SGLT2 inhibitor or alternative additional medications is usually made if the HbA1c blood test result is too high (that is, above 48 mmol/mol or 6.5 per cent). SGLT2 inhibitors can be associated with an increased risk of thrush or urinary infections; if these prove very troublesome, the medication must be stopped.

GLP1 analogues

The class of drugs known as GLP1 analogues is particularly good at helping people lose weight, and can be added to metformin if significant weight loss is required. Most must be given by injection (usually once a week) and, like metformin, they can be associated with side effects that affect the gut. Again, these are sometimes quite severe, and in such cases the drug should be stopped. The newest of these drugs is tirzepatide, which is both a GLP1 and also a GIP analogue and so has additional effects to reduce glucose levels and help weight loss.

DPP4 inhibitors

DPP4 inhibitors can be thought of as a weaker version of a GLP1 analogue, and in some people are effective at reducing glucose levels. They can be used instead of metformin or an SGLT2 inhibitor, if neither can be tolerated or used safely. They can also be added to these drugs to provide additional benefit if the HbA1c level remains too high. They are generally not prescribed with GLP1 analogues, as they work in a similar way.

Table 5.1. Common medications in current use for Type 2 diabetes.

Drug name	Brand name	How it is given	Side effects
Biguanide			
Metformin	Glucophage	Tablet 1–2× daily	Common: diarrhoea, bloating
SGLT2 inhibitors			
Canagliflozin	Invokana	Tablet 1× daily	Common: urinary infections, thrush Rare: ketoacidosis
Dapagliflozin	Forxiga		
Empagliflozin	Jardiance		
Ertugliflozin	Steglatro		

Drug name	Brand name	How it is given	Side effects
DPP4 inhibitors			
Alogliptin	Nesina	Tablet 1× daily	Rare: pancreatitis
Linagliptin	Trajenta		
Saxagliptin	Onglyza		
Sitagliptin	Januvia		
Vildagliptin	Galvus		
GLP1 analogues			
Exenetide	Byetta	Injection 2× daily	Common: reduced appetite, nausea, vomiting Rare: pancreatitis
	Bydureon	Injection 1× weekly	
Liraglutide	Victoza	Injection 1× daily	
Lixisenatide	Lyxumia	Injection 1× daily	
Dulaglutide	Trulicity	Injection 1× weekly	
Semaglutide	Ozempic	Injection 1× weekly	
	Rybelsus	Tablet 1× daily	
Tirzepatide (also activates GIP)	Mounjaro	Injection 1× weekly	
Sulfonylureas			
Glibenclamide	Daonil	Tablet 1× daily	Common: low blood glucose, weight gain Rare: abdominal pain, diarrhoea
Glimepiride	Amaryl	Tablet 1× daily	
Gliclazide	Diamicron	Tablet 1–2× daily	
Glipizide	Glucotrol	Tablet 1–2× daily	
Tolbutamide	Orinase	Tablet 2–3× daily	
Insulins			
Various types		Injection 1–4× daily	Common: low blood glucose, weight gain

Some people who have had Type 2 diabetes for many years may become deficient in insulin. In such situations, a sulfonylurea or insulin itself can be prescribed, usually in addition to other medications. I generally recommend avoiding these where possible, as they are usually associated with weight gain and increased insulin resistance, meaning that ever higher doses are required to control glucose levels.

Other drugs used for Type 2 diabetes include pioglitazone, acarbose and meglitinides (such as repaglinide). These are not included in this section as they are rarely used nowadays.

Reducing medications when managing Type 2 diabetes with lifestyle changes

As I said earlier, many health professionals, and people diagnosed with diabetes, see Type 2 diabetes as a condition that requires medication. While this is true for a percentage of those diagnosed, today there is increasing interest in managing the condition with lifestyle change. This interest has grown with the realisation that, in some cases, Type 2 diabetes can be reversed. If you choose to reverse your diabetes by eating a very low-calorie diet, then it is usually recommended that you stop all your diabetes medications when you start the low-calorie diet. This should be done under medical supervision since other medications, such as for blood pressure, may also need to be reduced. This approach is usually not recommended for people on insulin injections, although it is possible under close medical supervision.

If you follow the diet principles in this book – that is, avoid eating and drinking sugars and large portions of starchy foods – then it is important to ensure that, as you make changes to your diet, your blood glucose levels do not fall too low. If you take any medications, especially for diabetes or high blood pressure, then it is essential that you discuss your plan to change your diet with your doctor or diabetes nurse BEFORE you make any changes, as you may need to reduce some of your medications.

The top priority is to reduce medications that increase insulin in the circulation or cause weight gain, as these will prevent you being able to reverse the diabetes disease process. That means reducing the dose of any insulin or sulfonylurea that you are taking. My general advice is to halve the dose as you start to reduce your carbohydrate intake. These changes should be done after discussions with your doctor or diabetes nurse, especially if you are on more than one type of diabetes medication. As your glucose levels come down, you should be able to stop some or all these medications altogether.

If you are on one or more of metformin, SGLT2 inhibitor, DPP4 inhibitor or GLP1 analogue, then these can all be continued as you begin to reduce your carbohydrate intake. However, if you reduce your carbohydrate intake below 50 grams per day, then it is recommended that you stop taking SGLT2 inhibitors, because of the increased risk of diabetic ketoacidosis associated with a very low-carbohydrate diet. If you are taking an SGLT2 inhibitor for heart and kidney disease, then it is important that you seek medical advice before stopping it.

Other medications can then be reduced or stopped as your blood glucose levels fall. I generally suggest making a change if your fasting glucose is around 7 mmol/l (125 mg/dL) or less. My suggested order of doing this would be to stop taking your DPP4 inhibitor. Staying on a GLP1 analogue can be effective, particularly if you have a lot of weight to lose, as it helps to suppress appetite. However, that too can be stopped once you are well on your way to achieving your weight goal and/or your HbA1c is below 48 mmol/mol (6.5 per cent). The final drug to stop is metformin. Remember, if you can come off all your diabetes medications and maintain your HbA1c below 48 mmol/mol or 6.5 per cent, then by definition your diabetes is in remission. Remember also that if you revert to your previous eating pattern, your glucose levels will go up again, and you may need to restart medication. As Type 2 diabetes is a reversible condition, *remission is also reversible.*

Remember that any reduction in weight or HbA1c will benefit your health, even if you need to continue taking some medications. For example, if you lose weight and reduce your HbA1c to 45 mmol/mol or 6.3 per cent, but still need to take medications, this is by no means a failure. Quite the opposite!

Table 5.2 shows the medication changes that you should consider when starting a low-carbohydrate diet. I repeat, it is essential to discuss your medications with your GP or diabetes nurse before making any changes to your diet, as everyone has individual requirements that must be taken into account.

Other medications

A lot of people with Type 2 diabetes need to take medications for high blood pressure. This is because the high insulin levels that occur in people with Type 2 diabetes and prediabetes cause the body to retain more sodium (salt) in the blood. The high salt level means the body retains more water in the circulation (that is, in the blood), and that increases blood pressure. When you eat fewer carbohydrates, your insulin levels fall. This means that your salt levels fall, less water is in the circulation, and your blood pressure reduces. If you are on blood pressure medication, it is very important that you monitor your blood pressure using an automatic machine and, if necessary, reduce your blood pressure medications as your blood pressure falls. Please seek advice from your doctor or nurse about this.

Table 5.2. A guide to reducing or stopping medications.

Class of drug	Changes when starting a low-carbohydrate diet
Biguanide (metformin)	No change. Can be stopped if HbA1c is below 48 mmol/mol (6.5 per cent).
DPP4 inhibitors (e.g. sitagliptin)	No change initially. Can be stopped if fasting glucose levels fall below 7 mmol/l (125 mg/dL).
GLP1 analogues (e.g. liraglutide)	No change initially. Can be reduced and eventually stopped if fasting glucose levels fall below 7 mmol/l (125 mg/dL).
SGLT2 inhibitors (e.g. canagliflozin)	**Must be stopped if total carbohydrate intake is less than 50 grams per day.** Otherwise, it can be reduced and eventually stopped if fasting glucose levels fall below 7 mmol/l (125 mg/dL).
Sulfonylureas (e.g. gliclazide)	Halve the dose when starting a low-carbohydrate diet. Needs to be stopped if fasting glucose levels fall below 7 mmol/l (125 mg/dL).
Insulins (various types)	Generally, halve the dose when starting a low-carbohydrate diet. Doses can then be gradually reduced as glucose levels fall below 7 mmol/l (125 mg/ml). If glucose levels then begin to rise, revert to the previous dose and seek professional advice.
Blood pressure medications (various types)	Generally, reduce dose if systolic blood pressure is consistently less than 120.

As you lose weight and your blood glucose control improves, then you may find that other health problems (as well as high blood pressure) also begin to improve. I have known patients to come off medication for joint pain, acid reflux, gout and erectile dysfunction because they have adopted a low-carbohydrate diet. This is great for the individuals concerned, as well as for the National Health Service (NHS). It also shows how many health problems arise from being overweight or metabolically unhealthy.

Chapter 6

Losing weight the right way

Interventions to lose weight

For many people, eating a healthy diet and reducing their intake of sugars and other refined carbohydrates will lead to weight loss. Rather than set out strict rules to follow, my philosophy is to encourage each person to identify the *sustainable* changes they feel they can make, as they need to be able to live with these permanently. This might mean making one change at a time over a period of weeks or months. In that case, weight loss will be slower than when you go on a crash diet, but will be longer-lasting. If you want to lose more weight faster, then you have several options.

Reduce fat intake

Having said in Chapter 3 that I encourage you to reintroduce fat into your diet and not to count calories, it is important to be aware that fat is high in calories, and if you find you're eating a lot of nuts, cheese or other dairy products, this could be helping to reduce your glucose levels but might make it more difficult for you to lose weight. In this situation, I suggest you limit your intake of cheese and nuts.

Intermittent fasting/time-restricted eating

For the longest time fasting was considered unfashionable, often associated with religious observance or quackery. After all, haven't we all been told that we need three good meals a day? Well, we don't! Especially if we're overweight. There is a lot of evidence that fasting is very good for us in a variety of ways, especially if you want to lose weight. The key to losing weight if you have Type 2 diabetes is to reduce your insulin levels as much as you can. Reducing carbohydrates can certainly do that, but in some people, insulin levels remain too high, as protein in a meal can also increase insulin levels. One surefire way to reduce insulin levels is not to eat: in other words, to fast. The easiest way to do this is to skip breakfast on one or more days each week. By having a sixteen-hour overnight fast – from after your evening meal until lunch the following day – your insulin levels will plummet, and this helps you to burn off excess visceral fat and to lose weight.

Some people are simply not hungry in the mornings. If this is you, then you can save time and money by not eating breakfast! Others find they can manage it for one or two days each week, or more. I generally fast on days when I am busy – time flies and before I know it, it's time for an early lunch. Some people prefer to have a longer fast each week, for twenty-four or thirty-six hours. Again, what's important is that you find a routine that works for you. If you take insulin or sulfonylurea medication, then it is important to seek medical advice before fasting, as these medications will need to be reduced when fasting.

Very low-calorie diets

This is a very effective means of losing weight in a short period of time, and was the original intervention that showed that Type 2 diabetes could be reversed. It requires planning, as you may need to reduce or stop a number of medications, and you will need to have access to very low-calorie foods or supplements and a meal plan for several weeks. If you live in the UK and have recently been diagnosed with diabetes, you may be eligible to take part in the NHS Type 2 Diabetes

Path to Remission Programme.* People on this programme, which is free, are offered low-calorie, total diet replacement products, such as soups and shakes, for twelve weeks. They are also supported for twelve months, and helped to reintroduce food into their diets after the twelve-week meal-replacement programme.

Some people find this programme difficult to maintain; however, it can be done. The key is to ensure that when you come off the very low-calorie diet, you do not return to your old eating habits, as the weight can very easily pile back on. I therefore recommend that people who choose this approach change to a low-carbohydrate diet when they resume eating normally.

Other diets and eating plans

There are thousands of different weight loss diets available, and different people find different plans effective. I do not recommend any one in particular, but suggest that you avoid diets that include starchy carbohydrates, sugar and other ultra-processed foods in their eating plans. As always, your priority is to find a plan that suits your food preferences, does

* https://www.england.nhs.uk/diabetes/treatment-care/diabetes-remission/

not make you feel hungry, and that you feel you can continue in the long term.

Stopping smoking

We all know that smoking is bad for our health, and if you have Type 2 diabetes, the health risks from smoking are magnified by the effect of having diabetes. So it's important to stop smoking – and vaping – to protect your future health. It is also important to realise that it is very hard to change long-held habits, so it might be too much to expect for someone to stop smoking at the same time as giving up some of their favourite foods.

If you smoke, and you want to stop smoking, what is your priority? Is it to stop smoking, or is it to better manage your diabetes? If it is to stop smoking, then put your energies into stopping smoking first. If it is to reduce your glucose levels, then concentrate on making the dietary changes that will help you achieve that, and only start to think about stopping smoking once you have reached your initial lifestyle goals. In the UK, the NHS provides a range of initiatives to help people stop smoking; details are available at www.nhs.uk/better-health/quit-smoking.

Chapter 7

Monitoring your diabetes management

The aim of effective management of Type 2 diabetes is, first and foremost, to achieve near-normal levels of blood glucose as possible. For many people, this also requires them to lose weight, and to ensure their blood pressure is not elevated. As 99 per cent of all diabetes management is done by the person with diabetes, then it's essential that they have effective tools to monitor their progress and to show whether their chosen management strategy (for example, lifestyle changes and medications) are working. While it is true that diabetes clinics will monitor your weight, blood pressure, HbA1c and other blood tests, people attend these too infrequently for these to guide their diabetes management.

The tools that will help

Weighing scales

I recommend that you buy some good weighing scales, and that you weigh yourself on a regular basis – at least once a week. That is because body weight has such a big impact on glucose metabolism that you need to know if your weight is increasing so you can take corrective action to reduce it. Some people choose to weigh themselves every day. While this is not generally recommended, if this works best for you, and helps to reassure you, then carry on.

Blood pressure monitor

I also recommend that you buy an automated blood pressure monitor. The guidelines for measuring blood pressure recommend that you are seated and rested for five minutes before measuring blood pressure. I have not yet been to any medical facility that allows that. So often, blood pressure measurements in a clinic are higher than they would be at home. If you are not on any blood pressure medication and your blood pressure is within normal limits (i.e. below 140/85), then checking it once a month is enough. If you take blood pressure medication, and especially if you are making lifestyle changes, then I recommend checking your blood pressure at least once a week. This is important. With weight loss, your blood pressure is likely to reduce, meaning that you may need to reduce your blood pressure medication.

Blood glucose monitor

The most important way you monitor your diabetes management is by checking your blood glucose levels. This is the only way you can tell if the lifestyle changes you are making, and the medications you are taking, are having the desired effect. In the UK, many people with Type 2 diabetes are not provided with blood glucose monitoring equipment. It is recognised that glucose monitoring is essential for people who inject insulin, so they can monitor for low glucose levels. It is otherwise not considered essential that people know what their level is! I completely disagree with this policy. Thankfully, things are slowly changing, but many people are still not given any way to measure their blood glucose. If you are in this situation, then I recommend that you ask your GP to prescribe test strips for you, especially if you are planning to make lifestyle changes to better manage your diabetes. If they refuse, then you can buy strips online for about £25 for 100 strips. These will last a few months if used sparingly.

From Chapter 3, you know that what you eat has a huge impact on your blood glucose levels, so I recommend a form of testing called paired mealtime testing. This is where you check your blood glucose just before a meal, and then two to three hours afterwards. Ideally the glucose level should stay about the same, or rise at most by 2–3 mmol/l (30–50 mg/dL). You can use this information to adjust your diet – by reducing the carbs you eat in a meal – until the after-meal test result falls within the desired range. For example, if you have a portion of shepherd's pie with some green vegetables, and your glucose increases from 5 mmol/l (90 mg/dL) before the meal to 9 mmol/l (160 mg/dL) afterwards, then it is clear that something in the meal has pushed your glucose level up too high. This is most likely to be the potato in the pie. So the next time you have shepherd's pie, you could either have a much smaller amount of potato topping or use mashed celeriac instead – it has a much lower carbohydrate content. Once you have worked out the amount of carbohydrate that enables you to enjoy shepherd's pie without increasing your glucose levels, then as long as you keep to that amount, you will not need to do a test every time you eat that meal.

Paired tests

If you are just starting to make dietary changes, I suggest that you perform a paired test before and after a different meal each day. For example, breakfast on the first day, lunch the next day, then evening meal, and so on. It has been shown that performing a paired test before and after a meal six times a month can help people achieve better control of their diabetes.* Using tests in this way does not require a large number of test strips, so it's not very expensive.

Over time, as your body responds to the dietary changes you make, you should see that your glucose levels gradually come down towards normal. By definition, a normal fasting glucose level (taken first thing in the morning before any food or drink) is less than 6.1 mmol/l (110 mg/dL) and no higher than 7.8 mmol/ml (140 mg/dL) after a meal. If you have adopted a low-carbohydrate diet, then your level should be even lower after meals. A word of advice, however. It is generally considered that fasting glucose is the lowest over the day, and levels usually rise as they day progresses, unless you are on glucose-lowering medication. People who adopt a very low-carbohydrate ketogenic diet, however, may find that their fasting glucose is above 6.1 mmol/l (110 mg/dL) and sometimes as high as 7 mmol/l (125 mg/ml), and this may be worrying. This is a recognised phenomenon that is not completely understood. It is as if the body releases glucose in the early morning to prepare for the new day, but it has adapted to burning fat for its energy and so does not use the glucose, allowing the level in the blood to rise. This is likely a result

---

* Franciosi M, Lucisano G, Pellegrini F, et al. 'ROSES: role of self-monitoring of blood glucose and intensive education in patients with type 2 diabetes not receiving insulin: a pilot randomised clinical trial.' *Diabetic Med.*, 2011, 28: 789–96.

of being fat-adapted, and is probably a normal physiological response. I generally advise that if your fasting glucose is a bit high, but the level then falls for the rest of the day, and if your HbA1c is within the desired range, then there is no need to be concerned.

Continuous glucose monitoring systems

Over the past few years, non-invasive glucose monitoring systems have become available. These systems comprise a sensor, which is usually embedded in an adhesive patch on the skin, with a tiny cannula that sits just below the skin, which transmits the glucose level to a reader or an app on your phone. These continuous glucose monitoring (CGM) systems provide frequent readings of your glucose level without the need for repeated finger-prick testing. Earlier systems required a traditional blood glucose reading to be taken once a day to calibrate them and ensure they provide accurate readings, while more modern ones don't. It is important to be aware that these systems measure the glucose in interstitial fluid – that is, the fluid that surrounds the cells in the fat layer beneath the skin – rather than in the blood. There is usually a lag time of up to ten minutes between the two. If you are on insulin treatment, then this difference will be more relevant: you will need to know that if the sensor is reading low, your blood glucose level could be lower, or if the sensor is reading high, the level in your blood could be higher. This difference is rarely an issue in people with Type 2 diabetes.

The beauty of these systems is that they mean you can check your blood glucose at any time of day and night without having to do a finger-prick test. They also show you the exact impact of each meal on your glucose levels, and of other activities, such as going for a walk. I have no doubt that, in due course and as their cost comes down, these will become the standard means of monitoring for everyone with diabetes. In 2024, in the UK and many other countries, they are not routinely provided for people with Type 2 diabetes. However, their cost is already coming down, and a number of my patients with Type 2 diabetes have chosen to purchase a CGM system. The most widely used system in the UK is the FreeStyle Libre system manufactured by Abbott. Each sensor costs about £50 and lasts for two weeks, so the monthly cost is £100. It is clearly not cheap, but is within reach of many people. Some people use it all the time; others choose to use the system every few weeks. The glucose readings can be uploaded into the LibreView system, which allows your designated clinic or doctor to view your data and give you advice on any changes you need to make in the light of your glucose readings. If you can afford it, I recommend that you use a CGM system at least for a few months while you make lifestyle changes: it will be enormously helpful in guiding your food choices as you make changes to your diet. It is also hugely rewarding and motivating to see your levels come down as a result of your efforts.

There are a number of other systems becoming available. If you are interested in using such a system, I suggest you do your own research online to see what is out there.

Chapter 8

Alternative therapies and supplements

Alternative therapies

Yoga

I mentioned earlier that yoga is a form of exercise that can be recommended for people with Type 2 diabetes. A number of studies have shown that yoga is associated with improved health – and this includes improvements in Type 2 diabetes. Yoga has been shown to help reduce HbA1c, weight, cholesterol, blood pressure and cortisol (stress hormone) levels. A key aspect of yoga is relaxation, which would be expected to reduce levels of cortisol. This alone will have beneficial effects on glucose levels and body weight. I do not recommend yoga as the main treatment for diabetes, but if it is something you enjoy, then it may well help.

Acupuncture

Less easy to explain is the effect of acupuncture. I do not understand how it works, but a number of studies have shown that it can be associated with reductions in glucose levels. Again, I would not recommend it as your main treatment, but if you find it helpful, please use it.

Supplements

I am often asked about the best supplements for people with Type 2 diabetes. My usual answer is to try one for a period of time. If you feel it is helping to reduce your glucose levels, then continue with it. Some of the most-studied supplements include trace elements, vitamins and plant extracts.

Trace elements

The chemical element chromium is a steel-grey metal and a trace element in human bodies. It has been shown in several scientific studies to have an effect in reducing insulin resistance – a key goal in managing Type 2 diabetes. It is thought to play a role in helping insulin bind to its receptor on cell walls, which is the key (literally) to allowing glucose to enter cells. Chromium is found in foods such as meat, liver and whole grains (but most of the chromium is removed during the refining process in the production of white flour). A review of over forty studies* showed that supplements of chromium reduced glucose levels, and that the best effects were seen with chromium picolinate at doses of 400–1000 mcg (micrograms) a day. There is no evidence that chromium supplementation is harmful.

Studies have also shown beneficial effects of magnesium supplements in reducing insulin resistance and glucose levels. Zinc appears to increase insulin secretion, and may be useful in people who are deficient in insulin.

Vitamins

Vitamin D is more accurately described as a hormone. It helps the body maintain the correct level of calcium in the blood. For vitamin D to be effective, it needs to undergo a chemical change in the skin – and the catalyst for the change is sunlight. Adequate exposure to the sun is important to maintain vitamin D levels. Today, we spend most of our time indoors (or in the car). In the UK, chances of being able to expose our skin to sunlight are few and far between. It

---

* Balk E, et al. 'Effect of chromium supplementation on glucose metabolism and lipids: a systematic review of randomized controlled trials.' *Diabetes Care*, 2007, 30: 2154–63.

is hardly surprising, therefore, that vitamin D deficiency is quite a common problem and can be especially problematic in people with darker skin. A number of studies have suggested that a lack of vitamin D is associated with an increased risk of insulin resistance and Type 2 diabetes. Some studies* have shown that taking vitamin D can help reduce insulin resistance, while others have failed to show any benefit. Everyone is now advised to take vitamin D supplements in winter, and there is no harm in taking a small supplement of vitamin D (e.g. 25 mcg) daily, if only to reduce the risk of vitamin D deficiency and worsening insulin resistance that would cause.

It is often recommended to take vitamin K with vitamin D, and there is some evidence that vitamin K is effective in reducing HbA1c and insulin levels. In the liver, vitamin K acts to decrease insulin resistance.

Plant extracts

Cinnamon is obtained from the bark of trees from the *Cinnamomum* family, and has been used as a spice since biblical times. Studies have shown that a small dose (as little as

* Talaei A, Mohamadi M, Adgi Z. 'The effect of vitamin D on insulin resistance in patients with type 2 diabetes.' *Diabetol. Metab. Syndr.*, 2013, 5(1): 8.

1 g per day) of cinnamon cassia leads to a significant reduction in glucose and cholesterol levels. A review of several studies found that another variety (*Cinnamomum zeylanicum*) was associated with several changes.* Some nutritionists recommend that people with diabetes take 3 g (a teaspoonful) of cinnamon a day to help reduce their glucose levels, and some of my patients report benefit from taking it.

Berberine is an intensely yellow substance that is found in several plants, including Chinese goldthread and American goldthread. It has been shown to reduce insulin resistance.

Another plant supplement is psyllium husk, which derives from the Indian shrub *Plantago ovata*. It contains soluble fibre, forming a gel-like substance in the gut that can relieve constipation. It also delays food passing through the stomach, and can reduce the absorption of carbohydrate. Some people become constipated on a lower-carbohydrate diet, so taking psyllium husk can relieve this and help reduce glucose levels.

---

* Ranasinghe P, Jayawardana R, et al. 'Efficacy and safety of "true" cinnamon (*Cinnamomum zeylanicum*) as a pharmaceutical agent in diabetes: a systematic review and meta-analysis.' *Diabet. Med.*, 2012, 29(12): 1480–92.

Reducing stress

Even if we feel that our mental health is okay, many of us feel as though we're in a constant state of stress. We might not feel overtly stressed, but the way we live can lead to a state of low-level stress that is harmful to our health. Thirty years ago, for most people work started when they arrived at the workplace and ended when they left the workplace. Today, we now have the ability to send and receive emails on our mobile phones, we are always available, blurring the distinction between home and work time.

In many respects, these advances have been beneficial. We no longer have to wonder where anyone is as almost everyone has a personal tracking device, also known as a mobile phone. And yet, over the past thirty years, along with increasing rates of obesity and Type 2 diabetes, we have seen increases in a whole host of conditions, including depression, mood disturbances and chronic fatigue.

Cortisol is the body's main stress hormone. It increases whenever we are under any kind of stress. It increases our blood glucose levels and ratchets up the immune system as part of what is called the fight-or-flight response, to enable us to fight or run away from an enemy, and to help the body heal following any physical injury. These are all good things if we are in serious trouble – for example, if we're being attacked by a predatory wild animal, as would have happened to our ancestors. In such a situation, our cortisol level increases to help us survive the attack, then returns to normal base levels.

The problem is that, today, our body cannot readily distinguish between a real emergency and the multitude of stresses that impact our modern lives. As a result, any emotional, physical or mental stress can cause cortisol levels to spike – such as a serious illness, job or money worries, or being in an unhappy relationship. It could also be because we're rushing around doing one thing after another, or we're stuck in traffic and running late, or we receive a problematic email late at night. The net effect is that we're in a state of constantly high cortisol levels, meaning our immune system is constantly primed and our energy stores mobilised to prompt blood glucose levels to rise. It stands to reason that if your cortisol levels are constantly raised, it will make it very difficult to manage diabetes. Many people find that stress causes their blood glucose levels to rise significantly, even if they are following a healthy diet. Effectively managing stress is therefore essential – not just for your mental wellbeing, but also to help you manage your diabetes.

As we should eat more healthily to try to undo the harmful effect of unhealthy food, so we should do our best to undo the harmful effects of our hectic lifestyle on our bodies. Several things can help. One that is important and universally relevant is to take breaks during the working day. For years, working in a busy hospital, I would work for up to ten hours without stopping. I would grab a coffee during my clinic and take it back to my consultation room, and at lunchtime I would swallow a sandwich while checking emails. Very often, I would spend the entire day in one room. Then, about ten years ago, I attended a seminar in which we were shown brain activity scans of a person who had been sitting down for two hours, and the effect of a simple twenty-minute walk. The difference was incredible. After sitting down for a while, large parts of the brain had shut off – gone into 'sleep mode', as I described earlier in the book – yet after a short walk, the brain scan was lit up, metaphorically firing on all cylinders.

I now make it a habit to get out into the fresh air every morning. If I am at work, then I make a point of leaving the building and going out to buy a coffee. Unless it is pouring, I sit outside for a few minutes simply enjoying *being*, before returning to my clinic. A short break outside not only wakes up my brain and helps me become more alert to my patients' needs, but it also helps disrupt the constant state of stress I would otherwise exist in, reducing my cortisol levels and delivering all the benefits that come with that.

Many things happen in life that cause stress, and we cannot avoid all the situations that make us stressed, but we can learn to be more aware of how stress makes us feel and behave. I encourage you to think about what changes you can build into your daily routine that will reduce your risk of constantly feeling under stress. If you can recognise the symptoms, then you can take corrective action to reduce the effect of stress on your body. Part of that is to do something that many people consider selfish – doing something *just for you*.

Looking after yourself

In our busy world, where many of us have to juggle work and family responsibilities, it can be easy for us to forget to look after ourselves. Yet if you have Type 2 diabetes, it is essential that you make the effort to prioritise your health. Alongside improving physical health, it's important to look after our own mental wellbeing. We all need some 'me time'. A period on a regular basis just for you. And many of us are not good at this at all. I have witnessed many patients over the years prioritise the needs of their children, spouse or elderly parents over their own needs. And that can lead to becoming drained, exhausted and in a constant state of stress.

If you have a health condition that requires your attention, failing to attend to your own needs can seriously harm you. Looking after *you* is not being selfish. After all, if we don't value ourselves enough to cater for our own needs, then who will? And if anything happens to us, then those who depend on us will be left to fend for themselves. So, is there something that you would like to do, just for you, once or twice a week? It could be anything: an exercise class, learning a new skill, learning to play an instrument, or even sitting down in front of your favourite TV programme. The only thing that matters is that what you choose gives you pleasure.

The ultimate rest is sleep, and a good night's sleep is very important. All too often, however, we squeeze sleep in when we have finished our day's work and chores, regardless of when that is. Clients or colleagues may send us work emails right around the clock. What do you think is the effect of receiving a work email a short while before going to bed? At best, it might cause a few moments of stress. At worst, it will make you change your plans or stay up to deal with it . . . or lie awake worrying about it.

Social media is just one cause of disturbed sleep. We need to learn to respect our need for good-quality sleep. Poor sleep has a bigger impact on driving than drinking alcohol. Poor sleep also leads to increased levels of cortisol, and that increases appetite but decreases satiety – so you feel the need to eat more, yet still feel hungry. Even in people without diabetes, blood sugar levels are higher after a night of disturbed sleep, setting off the train of insulin resistance and fat storage, weight gain and Type 2 diabetes. Good sleep, on the other hand, has the opposite, beneficial effect.

In his book, *The 4 Pillar Plan: How to Relax, Eat, Move, Sleep Your Way to a Longer, Healthier Life*, Dr Rangan Chatterjee has a whole chapter on how to improve sleep, with many helpful tips. These include having ninety minutes of screen-free time before going to bed; aiming (where possible) to avoid mental stress or excessive exercise in the late evening; and sleeping in absolute darkness.

Section 3:

Living well with Type 2 diabetes

Chapter 9

The link between diabetes and mental wellbeing

From previous chapters, it will be evident that while a diagnosis of Type 2 diabetes can lead to serious health problems, there is a huge amount that you can do to prevent those problems happening, and even to improve your health now and in the future. However, that requires you to make permanent changes to what you eat, and possibly other aspects of your daily life. While these changes will bring benefits, change can create its own challenges. The diagnosis of diabetes and the changes you may need to make can also have an impact on your psychological health and on those around you. This chapter will describe some of those challenges and provide practical advice to help you and your loved ones live well with your diabetes.

Diabetes distress

Simply having Type 2 diabetes can be a cause of psychological ill health. The term 'diabetes distress' is used to describe the emotional and psychological effects experienced by people with diabetes. Diabetes distress is associated with higher glucose levels and increased risk of diabetes-related complications, and so it is important that it is taken seriously. There are a number of reasons why a person might develop diabetes distress. These include how they respond to being diagnosed with Type 2 diabetes, how they adjust to the lifestyle changes required to manage it, and how they cope with complications (if they arise). Even in the absence of long-term complications, just having high glucose levels can affect mood or the ability to concentrate, as well as cause unpleasant physical symptoms such as thirst, frequent urination and sexual dysfunction. These readily explain how diabetes can affect relationships and wellbeing. It is also easy to imagine how someone burdened by these problems might find it more difficult to make the necessary changes to their diet and lifestyle to manage their diabetes. It is not surprising, therefore, that diabetes distress is associated with being less physically active, having an unhealthy diet, and taking medications less regularly.

Mindset

The way people are treated when they are diagnosed with Type 2 diabetes creates a significant mental impression, and it may stay with them for many years. For many people, being diagnosed with diabetes comes as a nasty shock, and may be associated with a number of different emotions. Some of these powerful emotions can result from the thoughts, feelings and worries that naturally emerge when you are diagnosed with a health problem. Getting the right information at the beginning can help correct any misinformation that may lead to negative emotions. Until recently, even giving accurate information may still have caused negative emotions, as it was believed that Type 2 diabetes was permanent and over time would gradually and inevitably get worse. Put crudely, the message was 'You will have it for life, it will get gradually worse, but you can make changes that can slow down how quickly it gets worse.' I can easily understand why some people thought, 'Whatever I do won't make that much difference, so I might as well get on and enjoy myself.'

We now know that the Type 2 diabetes disease process can be reversed – and those who are newly diagnosed have the greatest chance of reversing the condition. Even if you have had diabetes for many years, you can make lifestyle changes that can partially reverse the condition, leading to better health, weight loss and better energy levels. Knowing that Type 2 diabetes can be reversed provides a message of hope and empowerment – the changes you make can, and will, help you improve your health. If conveyed correctly, I believe that this could lead to a lot less diabetes distress arising at the time of diagnosis.

Another source of diabetes distress arises from traditional advice about how diabetes should be managed, with its emphasis on medication rather than lifestyle, coupled with the conventional advice on diet that may make things worse. Both risk increasing feelings of helplessness. Focusing on prescribing medication can convey the message that it is the tablets that are the treatment, and can reduce a patient's desire to take control of their condition, especially if that medication leads to them putting on weight. A high-carbohydrate diet, which for many years was recommended for people with diabetes, risks causing high blood glucose levels, and further risks causing confusion and despondency in someone who believes they are doing 'the right thing'. My experience is that focusing on making lifestyle changes the main way of managing Type 2 diabetes, coupled with a simple explanation about which foods will help reduce blood glucose levels, helps people to feel that they are in control of their condition, and helps to reduce feelings of helplessness and of anxiety.

Depression

Apart from distress directly arising from having diabetes, there is a strong link between depression and Type 2 diabetes, with evidence that insulin resistance (as occurs in Type 2 diabetes) can affect the chemical balance in the brain and increase the likelihood of symptoms of depression. Unfortunately, we often use sweet foods as a pick-me-up if we are feeling down, stressed, or want to cheer ourselves up. Not only will this worsen the risk of diabetes, but sugar has a direct effect on the brain and causes a feeling of wellbeing – some people call it a sugar rush. Others describe getting sugar cravings as the effect wears off, leading them to eat more. A vicious cycle then is set in motion, where a person with insulin resistance is more liable to feeling depressed. They may then resort to eating sugary foods to improve their mood (which it does in the very short term), but that also worsens insulin resistance, which can lead to even lower mood, more sugar intake and so on. And as we know, as well as affecting mood, insulin resistance also increases body weight, blood glucose levels, and the risk of developing Type 2 diabetes.

The effects of diet

There is evidence that eating processed foods is associated with an increased risk of depression and mild cognitive impairment. Not only do sugar and other processed foods increase the risk of prediabetes and Type 2 diabetes, they also increase the risk of depression. There is, therefore, evidence of a circular causal link between an unhealthy diet and poor mental health. Poor mental health can lead to unhealthy eating, and an unhealthy diet can contribute to poor mental health. We also know that poor mental health can be associated with other unhealthy behaviours, such as being physically inactive.

So it is not surprising that people with Type 2 diabetes can experience higher levels of stress and depression. While that in itself sounds pretty depressing, the good news is that a healthier diet can improve mental health. A healthy diet of fresh, unprocessed foods, avoiding sugars and refined carbohydrates, will help to reduce insulin resistance and inflammation, improving both physical and mental health.

The power of exercise

Physical activity can also improve our mood. As I have already argued, one of the quickest (and cheapest) wins is to go out for a walk. A short walk can make us feel better, more alert and happier. Research has shown that simply being outside in nature improves health, including your mood, as nature has a calming effect on the brain. More intensive exercise – such as running, cycling or swimming – increases the production of endorphins by the hypothalamus and pituitary gland in response to pain or stress; this group of peptide hormones relieves pain and creates a general feeling of wellbeing.

Chapter 10

The impact of diabetes on relationships and family life

Now that we understand how Type 2 diabetes can impact mental health, you will be able to appreciate that it might have a knock-on effect on relationships and family life. But that's not the end of the story: diabetes can affect relationships and family life in many other ways.

Energy levels

Being part of a family is hard work at the best of times, especially if you have children at home or elderly relatives to care for. Having Type 2 diabetes can sap your energy for many reasons, and this can make it more difficult for you to attend to the demands of family and other relationships. Fatigue and low energy levels can occur if your glucose levels are high, or because of stress or depression, or due to disturbed sleep, as discussed below. Feeling tired can affect mood and lead to irritability, exacerbating relationship difficulties.

I had a patient who loved walking. It turned out that one of the biggest impacts of having diabetes was that she was no longer able to keep up with her husband on long hikes in the hills. Apart from making her feel bad about herself, this had a substantial and unexpected effect on an important aspect of her life with her husband. This spurred her on to make changes to her diet to lose weight and reduce her glucose levels. She was pleasantly surprised to see her energy levels improve so that she and her husband could once more enjoy their long walks, which helped to repair their relationship. It's a good example of how the many consequences of having diabetes are not necessarily permanent and can be improved with lifestyle changes.

Sleep

Poor sleep patterns are commonly found in people with diabetes. High blood glucose levels can cause sleep disturbance because of the need to get up to pee several times a night. Poor sleep exacerbates stress, which in turn leads to poor sleep. A good night's sleep requires a very low level of cortisol when you go to bed: stress, which increases cortisol, impairs sleep. A vicious cycle then develops when staying awake keeps cortisol levels up, affecting sleep, worsening insulin resistance and pushing up glucose levels. High glucose levels can also increase sleepiness. One female stands out in my mind: she told me that when her diabetes was first diagnosed, she was so tired that she often went to bed at 9 p.m. and wouldn't get up again until lunchtime. She would then fall asleep in her chair during the afternoon. As her glucose levels came down, her chronic tiredness improved and, in her words, she regained her 'awake life'.

Nerve pain as a result of diabetes can be exacerbated by high glucose levels. This can be particularly bad at night, and is therefore a further cause of disturbed sleep. Sometimes a simple painkiller such as paracetamol can help to ease the discomfort sufficiently to enable sleep.

People who are overweight can develop a condition called sleep apnoea, where excessive fat in the neck restricts the breathing passages, leading to breathing difficulties, and sometimes stopping breathing altogether for several seconds. Often it is the person's partner who is more aware of this condition, as the person themselves may not fully wake during the night, but the breathing problems still disrupt the quality of their sleep and they wake up feeling very tired. As a result, they can fall asleep easily during the day, and that can further disturb their night-time sleep rhythm. If you suffer from poor sleep, try to identify which of these factors could be causing it, and either take steps yourself, or seek medical help, to improve your sleep.

Concentration

Of course, poor sleep can lead to tiredness and poor concentration during the day. Concentration can also be affected by other factors related to diabetes that affect brain function. It has been shown that mild cognitive impairment is more common in people with raised glucose levels, insulin resistance, obesity and unhealthy eating patterns. It is often described as 'brain fog', where people find it difficult to concentrate or remember things. One of the clearest descriptions of brain fog that I have heard came from Tom Watson, former Member of Parliament in the UK and deputy leader of the Labour Party. In 2019, I attended a packed meeting in Parliament where he described the changes he experienced after losing 60 kg (132 pounds) in weight; apart from the obvious physical benefits, he spoke with great clarity about how his mind was sharper and his memory so much better than when he was heavier and had Type 2 diabetes. In his book *Downsizing*, he describes how he became more focused in meetings, could recall facts and figures without prompting, and felt much better prepared for speeches and interviews.

Tom also alludes to how, before he lost weight, he relied on his staff to enable him to function at the level expected for his position. His experience shows how symptoms can improve dramatically by effectively managing (or, in his case, reversing) Type 2 diabetes.

Food

Managing Type 2 diabetes effectively means you have to pay attention to what you eat and focus on eating foods that will help keep your glucose levels stable. It means avoiding foods that contain sugar as much as you can, and limiting starchy foods, as discussed in Chapter 3. Making such changes can be very difficult, and these difficulties can be made much worse if you live with, or work alongside, people who continue to eat the foods you are trying to avoid. Understandably, this can be a source of stress and conflict. There is plenty of evidence to suggest that making lifestyle and dietary changes are much easier if you have the active support of the people close to you. The 'office cake' culture can be all-pervasive; many people report how difficult it can be to resist cakes brought in by colleagues.

The truth is, reducing sugar and other refined carbohydrates is likely to be beneficial for *everyone* – so ideally, your family will come on board by making some changes to their diet, so you can continue to share meals. If this is not possible, then at least ask them to help you by not flaunting their chocolate biscuits, breakfast cereals and other sweet (or savoury) treats, thereby leading you into temptation.

Routines

Managing Type 2 diabetes can affect other aspects of daily life that could impact family relationships. Although people with diabetes are no longer advised to eat at set times, if you take insulin or sulfonylureas then you may need to keep to a routine of eating at certain times, and this may conflict with what others in your household are doing. If this is the case, then it might be possible to make changes to your treatment so that this is not necessary. If you choose to reduce your meal frequency by not having breakfast, this should not impact those around you, but changes to your lunch or evening meals might do so, and it will be important to bear this in mind as you consider how best to manage your diabetes.

Sex

You now know that Type 2 diabetes can lead to a lot of physical and mental symptoms, and these, along with its effects on mood, can be a real dampener when it comes to sexual function and intimacy. In addition, high glucose levels can directly impair the function of nerves that are required for sexual arousal and function in both men and women. There used to be a taboo around discussing these problems, but with the arrival of Viagra in the late 1990s, discussion about erectile dysfunction has become normalised; treatments are regularly advertised on TV and are available without prescription.

Unfortunately, women's sexual problems remain largely ignored. This is partly because treatment options are limited to lubricants to combat dryness, or oestrogen creams to counter some of the effects of the menopause. While some early studies suggested that drugs such as Viagra can help some aspects of female sexual function, none has been proven to make a significant difference.

Living with Type 2 diabetes poses a lot of challenges to personal and family relationships. My aim in listing them here is to enable you to recognise how having diabetes can impact relationships, and to encourage you to have open discussions with loved ones or work colleagues about how having diabetes affects you, and how they can help you to deal with it.

Managing special occasions

Adapting your diet to manage diabetes is no picnic (apologies), and can be difficult at the best of times, but once you get used to it, it becomes part of your daily routine. This is fine when you are having a 'routine' day, but what can you do when you find yourself outside your normal routine – eating out, attending a special occasion or travelling?

You can never be sure what is in your meal when eating out, but you can make your life easier by choosing lower-carbohydrate options from the menu: avoid pizzas, pastas and pies, for example. Many restaurants will swap items so you can ask for extra vegetables or salad instead of potatoes or chips. Increasingly, waiting staff ask if you have any food allergies. Take them at their word and use this as an opportunity to specify your need for a meal that is free of sugar and low in carbohydrate. With a bit of trial and error, you should be able to identify cafes and restaurants near to you that make it easier for you to manage your diabetes without ruining what should be an enjoyable experience. Similarly, when you are invited to eat at a friend's house, learn to explain politely that you need to avoid sugar and large portions of starchy food.

Special occasions such as parties, weddings or other functions can be more of a challenge, as you will likely have less control over what is available to eat. Many buffets are very starchy, and the low-carb options may be limited to a few sad, limp pieces of salad garnish. Some people eat before such functions so they do not go hungry, as they expect there will be little they will be able to eat there, or use it as an opportunity to miss a meal (see the 'Intermittent fasting/time-restricted eating' section on page 94). Sometimes you may have no option but to eat what is on offer. If that is the case, as long as you keep away from high-sugar foods, then enjoy what you can, accept that your glucose level will go high for a while, but be reassured that this will not cause you any lasting problems.

Travel poses similar challenges. Most food available at railway stations and airports is starchy, so plan ahead and go to a supermarket to buy lower-carb options to take with you. It will also be much cheaper! Most holiday destinations in southern Europe will offer good low-carb options – the legendary Mediterranean diet is, after all, claimed to be one of the most healthy eating patterns. The USA – home of fast food – and central Europe can be more challenging. I recently visited Germany, where restaurant meals were very heavily based on meat and potato, dumplings or pasta in various forms. If you find yourself in this situation, you may have to eat foods you would usually avoid – however, if you can, try to substitute the starchy food for a salad.

Talking about your health

Since diabetes can impact many facets of personal and work life and relationships, it is important to feel comfortable talking about your health in an appropriate way. I am sure we all know some people who speak incessantly about their health problems, whereas others just get on with their life and barely mention their health, even if they have significant issues. Neither extreme is ideal, so what is an appropriate way to speak about your health?

I encourage you to be open about your health and to learn how to talk to people about it. This doesn't mean you need to divulge personal information, or bore everyone with every detail of your diabetes journey. But I regard it as healthy to be able to express your needs, especially around your diet, and explain how those around you can help you manage your condition – by, for example, not offering you sweet foods.

Don't blame yourself

Some people find it difficult to talk about their health, especially if they feel there is a certain stigma, and even shame, around Type 2 diabetes – as if they are responsible for bringing it on themselves. If people feel like this, they will not discuss their health at all, or they may even try to conceal the fact that they have diabetes.

I'd like to address this head-on. The number of people with Type 2 diabetes across the globe has increased by over 400 million in the past twenty years. Now, these people haven't all suddenly decided to eat unhealthy foods and laze around all day getting fat. However, like every creature in nature, they have consumed the food in their immediate environment, which has changed out of all recognition in just a few decades. This includes a huge range of ultra-processed foods that are designed to be extra tasty and to make us want to eat more, with the aim not of providing nourishment but of maximising the manufacturer's profits. So in a sense you are the victim, not the perpetrator – and it is to your credit that you are determined to do something about it, to revert to eating natural and healthy foods.

For most people, an important reason to talk about their diabetes is so that people understand *why* they cannot do or eat certain things, or to explain why they might be experiencing certain symptoms. Not everyone needs to know that you have diabetes, but if the people you spend most time with know, then it will be easier for you to mention it when you need someone else to know that it is affecting you in some way. For people who are naturally private about their health, this could be a big ask. If so, it might be easier to send a quick text or email to people who need to know, along the lines of: 'Just to let you know, I have Type 2 diabetes. This means I need to change my diet in certain ways and do some things differently. I'll try not to let it affect me too much, but please bear with me as I make adjustments.' Then if you are invited round for a meal, that doesn't have to be the first time you mention your diabetes; instead, you can mention your dietary requirements. In particular, the British can be overly polite and will eat something that is bad for their health rather than offend the host, so it's not a bad idea to practise how you can say, politely but firmly: 'Thanks, but no thanks. I can't eat that because it's bad for my health.' Or: 'Please would you *not* bring cakes into my office, as I can't eat them.' Or: 'Please don't offer me sweet biscuits. They will push up my sugar level and make me feel unwell.' Or when you are invited out for a meal, you could tell your host that, while you are very much looking forward to the meal, 'I know you'll understand that I can't eat large amounts of starchy food or sweet desserts!'

The people most likely to be affected by your diabetes, and who will potentially have most impact on your diabetes, are, of course, the people you live with, buy food with and share meals with. Hopefully, they will be on your side and will support you to manage your diabetes, or will help you manage some of the effects of having diabetes. But they can only do that if they *understand* what that means in practice. So do explain to them what your needs are, and how they can help you – politely, calmly and without apportioning blame. There may be times when it will be helpful for someone around you to know how you are feeling – for example, if your glucose level is very high – so they can understand why you might be a bit short-tempered, or repeatedly dashing to the loo. Whatever it is, establish and keep to hand a set of practised, polite phrases that will enable people to understand your situation and/or needs.

Some people find it helps to bring their spouse or partner to clinic visits, especially when they will be discussing a symptom of their diabetes that they find troublesome or worrying. When food and/or other lifestyle factors are being discussed, very often the changes the person with diabetes wishes to make will benefit their partner too!

Chapter 11

Supporting a person with diabetes

In Chapter 10, we discussed several ways in which having diabetes can impact those around you. Managing your diabetes can be much easier if you have a partner or friend willing and able to support you as you try to change your lifestyle. This chapter is written for them. After you have read this chapter, do ask those close to you to read it as well. It will show them how best they can help you.

Information for family and friends

If you live with, or care for, someone with diabetes, then you will be aware of the many demands that the condition places on that individual, and probably on you too. The aim of this book is to help those with Type 2 diabetes more effectively manage their condition, so they can maximise their health and reduce the likelihood of their diabetes causing further health problems in the future. They might even be able to reverse the disease processes that cause diabetes.

Until recently, it was believed that once you developed Type 2 diabetes, it was a progressive condition that simply got worse over time and it was a condition the person would have for life. But now we know that Type 2 diabetes results from excess fat accumulating in the liver and the pancreas, and that by making dietary changes this fat can be reduced, which helps to reverse the diabetes disease process. In many cases this enables the person with Type 2 diabetes to achieve lower blood glucose levels, reduce their medication, and lose weight. In some cases, their Type 2 diabetes goes into remission – although it will reappear if they revert to their previous eating habits.

The main problem in Type 2 diabetes is that the body cannot use insulin properly. This leads to the pancreas producing extra insulin, resulting in the levels of insulin in the blood rising too high. As insulin is the main 'fat hormone', the high insulin level leads to more fat being laid down in the internal organs, which makes the problem even worse.

We know that making lifestyle changes and losing weight can help reduce insulin levels. The most important change that needs to be made is to the diet. Specifically, it is essential to try to cut out sugar – in all its forms – as much as possible. Sugary drinks, such as fizzy drinks or sodas, fruit juices and smoothies, are particularly bad as they all cause the level of sugar in the blood to rise, leading the body to produce a large amount of insulin. It is also important to try to cut out sweet treats (such as biscuits, sweets and cake) and even sweet fruits (such as pineapple, banana and dried fruit).

The other main change is to reduce the amounts of starchy foods eaten, which includes bread and other flour-containing products: pasta, rice, potatoes and cereals. The reason is that all these are turned into glucose in the body, pushing up the levels in the blood and causing insulin to be released into the bloodstream. Reducing sugars and starches helps by keeping the blood glucose level stable, avoiding high insulin levels. Over time, as insulin levels reduce, the amount of fat in the liver reduces. Insulin can then again work more efficiently to control sugar levels, which in turn means the body does not release so much of it into the bloodstream, leading to a virtuous circle of positive health benefits.

The other recommended changes to eating patterns include only eating when hungry and avoiding snacks as much as possible. So, if an individual is not hungry in the mornings, there is no need for them to eat breakfast. In fact, having a long overnight fast until lunchtime is a really good way of burning excess fat. In the same way, not snacking between meals helps keep glucose and insulin levels lower for more of the day.

I realise that this may not be what you were told in the past. You may have been told that people with diabetes should eat starchy carbohydrates with every meal, and in some cases they should also snack in between meals. But that approach has not worked, whereas more and more people, including many I have treated, have found that restricting carbohydrates really does work.

In many countries, diets have changed significantly in recent years, with ready meals, fast food, takeaways and huge portions becoming the norm. That is one reason why so many people are becoming overweight and developing Type 2 diabetes. So, to reverse the diabetes disease process and to help people better manage their diabetes, it is essential to revert to the type of diet our parents or grandparents ate – based on fresh, real foods.

For many people, this will mark a significant change in their eating habits. The majority of us find change difficult, and it is enormously helpful if other people in the household, or the workplace, respect the changes the individual is trying to make, and supports them in their efforts. Anyone will find it easier to avoid eating biscuits and cakes if others agree not to bring them into work or home – or, if they do, to be discreet and not eat them openly. It can help to have lower-carbohydrate alternatives (such as vegetable sticks or small portions of cheese or nuts) readily available instead.

It is important that the person with diabetes sets their own goals and decides the pace at which *they* want to make changes. It is also important to be realistic: sometimes life throws a spanner in the works, sometimes people find it hard to maintain the changes, and this might lead them to go off track. In this situation, they will find it incredibly helpful to have someone who can support them and encourage them to get back on track. Many people with diabetes think that they also need to exercise. While exercise has many benefits, I encourage people to focus on changing their diet first, as this will have the biggest benefit. Increasing walking as part of their daily routine and breaking up sedentary (sitting down) periods is enough in the early stages.

In my clinic, I have seen that people do so much better when their partner or a close friend supports them, especially when they join them by making the same lifestyle changes. And in many cases their own health improves as well, which can't be a bad thing!

Diabetes can affect people in so many ways, as explained in Chapter 10 of this book. This includes having low energy levels or being irritable due to changing blood glucose levels. These could get worse in the short term as changing routines can in itself be stressful. Knowing that this could happen and having strategies in place to deal with any setbacks will help; this is covered in more detail in Chapter 12.

I am sure that the person who asked you to read this will be very grateful for your help in supporting them to make these changes so, on behalf of them – a big 'thank you' for any help you can offer as they make changes to manage their diabetes.

Chapter 12

Moving forward

Monitoring progress

Lifestyle changes are a significant part of managing your diabetes. Since you are the person in charge of your lifestyle, it is important that you have some way of monitoring your progress towards your goals. For many people, losing weight is an important goal. I strongly recommend that you invest in a good set of weighing scales. Digital scales are often easier to read. It makes sense to weigh yourself at the same time of day, perhaps first thing in the morning, naked, before you have eaten anything and after you have been to the toilet. Remember that a full stomach or bladder and wearing clothes will all increase your weight. I suggest you weigh yourself once a week – although some people like to weigh themselves every day as part of their routine – but the main thing is that you weigh yourself regularly. This helps you identify whether you are losing weight or not. Seeing that you are on track can be highly motivating. If you find that you are not losing weight, this should prompt you to review what you are doing and to seek further advice if needed (we cover steps you can take in this situation in Chapter 13).

Another very useful way of monitoring your progress is to measure your waist. Your lifestyle changes are designed to help you lose excess fat in your abdomen so, as that fat reduces, your waist will shrink. One of the most common 'complaints' I hear in my clinic is that patients have to buy new trousers! Using a tape measure, measure across the widest part of your abdomen – usually at the level of your tummy button. When measuring, ensure that the tape measure is not too tight: take the measurement after you have gently exhaled. Many people find that their waist is shrinking, even if they have not lost much weight.

If you have chosen to set yourself a goal of reducing your blood glucose from a high level, consider setting an interim goal. If your fasting glucose is generally between 15 and 20 mmol/l (270–360 mg/dL), perhaps set a goal to achieve a level of 10 mmol/l (180 mg/dL) in the first instance. Measure your fasting glucose at least once a week so you can track your progress towards your goal. Measuring just before and two hours after a meal every day will help you monitor the impact of what you eat, and will help you adjust what you eat so you can aim to only eat foods that do not push up your glucose level. If you can afford it, I recommend purchasing glucose sensors such as the FreeStyle Libre (see page 105) and using them for a few months so you can track your glucose levels – and the impact of the meals you eat – every day.

What medical checks do you need?

Once you have been diagnosed with Type 2 diabetes, it is important to go for regular health checks, to assess whether you have any signs of impending complications that might need treatment. If you manage to put your diabetes into remission, then I still advise you to have these checks, to ensure all remains well.

In the UK, the NHS has identified nine key care processes that everyone with diabetes is entitled to, and should receive, on an annual basis. They are shown in Table 12.1. Health systems in other countries will have similar recommendations, but since healthcare in many countries is within the private sector, it is often left to the person with diabetes to access (and pay for) these services.

Table 12.1. Nine annual care processes for people with diabetes.

Responsibility of diabetes care providers	
1. HbA1c (blood test for glucose control)	**5. Urine albumin-to-creatinine ratio** (urine test for risk of kidney disease)
2. Blood pressure (measurement for cardiovascular risk)	**6. Foot risk surveillance** (examination for foot ulcer risk)
3. Serum cholesterol (blood test for cardiovascular risk)	**7. Body mass index** (measurement for cardiovascular risk)
4. Serum creatinine** (blood test for kidney function)	**8. Smoking history** (question for cardiovascular risk)
Responsibility of NHS Diabetes Eye Screening	
9. Digital retinal screening (photographic eye test for early detection of eye disease)	

These are simple tests or measurements that monitor your health; they do not do anything to actually improve it. However, in the UK in 2021–22, less than 30 per cent of people aged under forty received the basic nine care processes; this increased to 35 per cent for people between forty and fifty-nine, and to just over 40 per cent for people over sixty. It is likely that care aimed at helping people manage their diabetes is even less readily available. That has certainly been my experience, especially since the Covid-19 pandemic, when the UK primary care system has been so overstretched that some patients find it difficult to access basic care.

If you find yourself in this situation, I encourage to take the initiative and ask your GP practice to arrange the key checks and give you feedback on the results. If you sign up for the NHS app, you can access this information via the app. In many other countries, results are sent direct to the patient. The next section describes the nine recommended care processes in turn, why they are necessary, and – where appropriate – what you can do if your test result is not as it should be.

1. HbA1c

This was described in detail in Chapter 1. In essence, it is a simple blood test that provides an overview of your blood glucose levels over the past two to three months. For management of Type 2 diabetes, the current NICE guidelines recommend that treatment should be directed to achieve an HbA1c of 48 mmol/mol or 6.5 per cent, except for people on treatment with insulin or a sulfonylurea tablet, when the target is higher (53 mmol/mol or 7 per cent) to reduce the risk of abnormally low glucose levels. For anyone who wants to achieve remission of their diabetes, a level of below 48 mmol/mol (6.5 per cent) without any diabetes medication is required.

2. Blood pressure

Blood pressure is the level of pressure that the blood is under in blood vessels. The cells that make up the body need glucose and oxygen (plus a huge number of other substances) to function effectively. Blood carries these necessary chemicals and nutrients to every part of the body. For blood to function effectively, it needs nice clean blood vessels to flow through and it needs to be under pressure in order to flow (against the force of gravity a lot of the time). Blood pressure comes primarily from the action of the heart, the specialised muscle that acts as a pump to squeeze blood through the arteries. The kidneys also have an important role in controlling blood pressure, by producing hormones that help control how tightly the blood vessels contract (to increase pressure) or relax (to reduce blood pressure). The kidneys also regulate blood pressure by controlling the amount of water and salt in blood vessels. It will be obvious that diseases of either the heart or the kidneys may cause problems with blood pressure regulation – and can make an existing blood pressure problem worse.

One of the roles of insulin is to act on the kidneys to retain water and salt. Therefore, high insulin levels will keep more water and salt in the circulation, directly increasing blood pressure. This explains why people with Type 2 diabetes and prediabetes are more likely to have high blood pressure. A vicious circle can then develop: having Type 2 diabetes increases the risk of high blood pressure; this combination can lead to heart and kidney problems, which can then make the blood pressure problem worse. High blood pressure increases the risk of further complications such as a stroke or heart attack, and so it is essential that blood pressure is closely monitored in everyone with Type 2 diabetes.

Blood pressure is measured using a machine connected to a cuff that is placed tightly around the upper arm. The machine causes the cuff to inflate until the pressure it exerts around the arm is high enough to stop the blood flowing through the main artery, called the brachial artery. The cuff pressure is then gradually decreased until the blood flow returns to normal. As it does, a sensor detects when the cuff reaches the level of the pressure in the arteries as the heart is contracting (called systolic blood pressure) and the level of the pressure as the heart is relaxing (called diastolic blood pressure). These results are then displayed on a digital display as two numbers, with the systolic pressure first: for example, 120/80. The actual numbers refer to millimetres of mercury (mm Hg), relating back to the days of manual machines that had a column of mercury in them, like a thermometer.

There are many guidelines that specify the ideal blood pressures in different circumstances, but as a general rule it should be below 140/85. If you have evidence of kidney or eye disease, then a lower level may be recommended. Just like blood glucose, blood pressure levels vary quite considerably during the day, according to what you are doing and experiencing. Just as a single blood glucose measurement cannot give an accurate overview of your diabetes control, neither can a single blood pressure measurement be used to determine your blood pressure control.

Ideally, blood pressure should be measured in a relaxed environment after resting for at least five minutes, yet it is often measured in a busy clinic setting, perhaps after you have been waiting for some time, getting more and more tense. I therefore recommend that everyone with diabetes buys a machine to do measurements at home. I recommend not using one that wraps around your wrist like a watch, as these can be less accurate. You can buy one that has a cuff to wrap around the upper arm for £30 or less. I suggest checking your blood pressure no more than once every two weeks – just to reassure yourself (and your doctor) that all is well. If your blood pressure is high, or you are on medication for blood pressure, then more frequent monitoring may be required. If your blood pressure has been found to be consistently high, then it is important to try to reduce it. You may need tablets to achieve this, but lifestyle changes should also help.

If you follow the dietary changes I recommend in this book, you will likely reduce your blood insulin levels, and this should help reduce your blood pressure as well. Stress can also increase blood pressure, so managing stress (as discussed in Chapter 8), will also help keep blood pressure under control.

3. Serum cholesterol (blood test)

Cholesterol has received a lot of bad press in recent years and has been blamed for all manner of ills. However, the body needs cholesterol for many functions. Cell membranes, which control what enters your body's cells, are largely made of cholesterol. Vitamin D, which is essential for healthy bones, and many hormones are also made from cholesterol. So, cholesterol is important.

However, many of us have high levels of cholesterol in our bloodstream. High levels of cholesterol have been shown to be associated with cardiovascular disease, such as heart attacks and strokes. It has also been shown that eating a diet high in saturated fat increases cholesterol levels. This led to the belief that, since eating saturated fat increases cholesterol levels, and as high cholesterol increases the risk of cardiovascular disease, eating saturated fat must increase the risk of heart disease. This belief has since been challenged. It is perhaps more likely that high insulin levels (as in insulin resistance and Type 2 diabetes) lead to both high cholesterol levels and an increased risk of heart disease. For a long time, we have known that not all cholesterol is bad. It is the balance of the different types of cholesterol that is important, rather than the total number. There are two main types of cholesterol, LDL (low-density lipoprotein) cholesterol (generally thought of as bad for us) and HDL (high-density lipoprotein) cholesterol, generally thought of as healthy. There is another type of fat called triglycerides, which is also generally accepted to be harmful. It is a fat in the blood, typically increased by eating carbohydrates or by alcohol.

As a rule, your cholesterol levels should be as follows:

Total cholesterol below 5 mmol/l (190 mg/dL)
LDL cholesterol below 3 mmol/l (115 mg/dL)
HDL cholesterol above 1 mmol/l (40 mg/dL) in men; 1.2 mmol/l (45 mg/dL) in women
Triglycerides below 1.7 mmol/l (150 mg/dL)
Total chol:HDL ratio below 4
Trig:HDL ratio below 2

The pattern most associated with heart disease is a low HDL cholesterol and a high triglyceride level. Therefore, if you have a high HDL cholesterol and low triglyceride level, you are likely to have a reduced risk of heart disease, even if your total cholesterol level is high (because of the high HDL level). Moreover, there is some evidence to suggest that this applies even if you have a high level of LDL cholesterol. That is why risk calculators such as QRISK3 (which estimate a person's risk of cardiovascular disease) use the ratio between total and HDL cholesterol rather than the absolute numbers.

The NICE guidelines suggest that people with Type 2 diabetes should be offered treatment with a statin if their QRISK assessment suggests they have a 10 per cent or greater risk of developing cardiovascular disease over the next ten years. You can calculate your risk at https://qrisk.org/index.php. This tool uses your HDL and total cholesterol levels to calculate your risk. If your HDL is too low, and consequently increases your risk, you may wish to have the test repeated a few months after you have made lifestyle changes to reduce your overall risk, rather than take a statin. The good news is that the same changes that help reduce your blood glucose and blood pressure will also help your cholesterol level. So, increasing your physical activity, eating a healthy diet and losing weight will all contribute to improving cholesterol levels. And beware of being taken in by low-fat foods, or foods that claim to reduce cholesterol levels. While there may seem to be a certain logic in saying that eating less fat will reduce your cholesterol level, remember that insulin is the main fat-producing hormone, so reducing your carbohydrate intake will help reduce your insulin level. That will, in turn, enable you to lose weight.

Statins are drugs that work by reducing the amount of cholesterol released from the liver into the bloodstream. They are undoubtedly effective in reducing cholesterol levels, and only need to be taken once a day. However, they can cause side effects, particularly when used at higher doses. The most common side effect is the reported incidence of muscle aches and pains; sometimes this can be associated with a potentially serious inflammation of the muscles known as myositis. However, as statins have become more widely used, a number of other side effects have been reported, such as headaches, difficulty in sleeping, joint pains and poor concentration. If you experience a new symptom since taking a statin, my advice would be to stop the statin for a few weeks. Generally, if the symptom is related to the statin, it will soon disappear after stopping the medication. You may be able to manage better with a lower dose of the statin, or with a different statin. Occasionally alternative types of medication may be required.

Some people feel strongly that they do not wish to take a statin. This is a personal choice, and it is of course each person's right to decide whether they wish to take a particular treatment. My approach is to assess everyone according to their situation. If you have had a heart attack, are overweight and have high blood pressure, then taking a statin is likely to protect your health in the future. If, on the other hand, you have no history of cardiovascular disease, have lost weight and your blood pressure is normal, then it is likely that a statin will only have a small overall benefit.

Just as with high blood pressure, there are no symptoms associated with having a high cholesterol level, so it is important to have a blood test done once every year to check your cholesterol levels.

4. Serum creatinine (blood test)

The creatinine blood test is used to determine the estimated glomerular filtration rate (or eGFR) and is a measure of kidney function. Creatinine is a by-product of the body's breakdown of protein, and is excreted by the kidneys. If the kidneys are not working properly, creatinine is not excreted into the urine and consequently the amount of creatinine in the blood accumulates. A normal eGFR is generally over 90, although many people may have an eGFR below this. A level below 60, however, indicates some impairment of kidney function and should be investigated, usually with a scan of your kidneys and other blood tests.

5. Urine albumin-to-creatinine ratio

The other test of kidney function is a urine test to assess the amount of a protein called albumin in the urine. Albumin is a protein in the blood. While the kidneys should normally excrete creatinine into urine, there should only be a very small amount of albumin in urine. However, in diabetic kidney disease the blood capillaries become leaky, which means that substances such as albumin leak through into the urine. This provides a simple way to check whether the kidneys are working properly. For this test, you need to provide a sample of urine. It is sent to a laboratory to have the level of albumin and of creatinine measured. The result is expressed as the albumin-to-creatinine ratio (or ACR for short). A level of up to 3 is generally considered normal. If your test result is higher than this, it does not mean that you have diabetic kidney disease, as other factors may cause a higher level (for example, a urinary infection or increased physical activity). If the result is above 3, then two further urine samples should be taken first thing in the morning. Very often these will be normal: however, if the levels are consistently raised then this suggests that your kidneys have been affected by diabetes. A slightly raised level (e.g. up to 30) is termed 'microalbuminuria' (literally, 'small amount of albumin in the urine') and is treated with medication to reduce the pressure in the kidneys. The usual treatment is an ACE inhibitor, such as ramipril, which is also used to treat high blood pressure. Increasingly, SGLT2 inhibitor tablets (see Chapter 5), which reduce blood glucose levels, are also used to protect kidneys from further damage. These treatments, together with better control of glucose and blood pressure, can help reduce the albumin leak, sometimes to normal levels.

Higher levels of ACR are termed macroalbuminuria. This will also require treatment with an ACE inhibitor and an SGLT2 inhibitor. These might not improve the albumin leak but will usually prevent further damage. Without treatment, however, diabetic kidney disease can progress to cause scarring of the kidneys, high blood pressure and eventually kidney failure. Fortunately, this is now rare in people with Type 2 diabetes. However, if you have albumin in your urine, you will have no symptoms to warn you of this, so – as with the other checks in this chapter – it is vitally important to have regular urine tests done, so that if there is evidence of diabetes affecting your kidneys, appropriate treatment can be started to prevent more serious damage.

6. Foot risk surveillance

Just as regular eye examinations are important, regular foot examination is a key part of diabetes care. Feet can be affected both by diabetic nerve disease – causing numbness and loss of sensation in your feet – and by blood vessel disease (which reduces blood flow). It is therefore important that your feet are examined on a regular basis (at least once a year). The examination is relatively straightforward and includes a check on the pulses in the feet (preferably using a Doppler machine, which assesses the flow through the arteries) and a simple check to test sensation. A nylon fibre (called a monofilament) is used to touch the sole of the feet in specific areas to see if you can feel it. The tests may pick up problems before you are aware of them. If they do, this should prompt a review of your diabetes management to ensure that everything is being done to minimise any further damage. A minor reduction in blood flow can be improved by increasing leg exercise such as walking; a more severe reduction can be further investigated by more detailed scans of the arteries. If these show evidence of narrowing or blockage, then surgery can help to improve blood flow. Loss of sensation is usually due to high glucose in the blood affecting the sensory nerves, and stabilising this can sometimes improve nerve function.

7. Body mass index

Body mass index (or BMI) is a calculation to determine if you are overweight for your height. Normal body weight is defined as having a body mass index between 20 and 25. A BMI between 25 and 30 is defined as overweight, and above 30 as obese. The precise calculation is to take the weight in kilograms and to divide it by the square of the height in metres. So for a person who weighs 80 kilos (about 12.5 stone) and is 1.83 m tall (about 6 feet), the BMI is calculated as:

$$80/(1.83 \times 1.83) = 23.9$$

This is in the normal range.

A person of the same height who weighs 110 kilos (about 17 stone) has a BMI of $110/(1.83 \times 1.83) = 32.9$ (which is in the obese range). A BMI calculator is available at https://www.nhs.uk/health-assessment-tools/calculate-your-body-mass-index/.

The BMI is an imprecise measure, and it needs to be interpreted with caution. A bodybuilder with very big muscles could have a high BMI, as muscle is much heavier than fat, and so it is quite possible for someone to be 'overweight' but in reality to be fit and healthy. Some experts suggest that waist circumference is a better measure of obesity, as most people who are genuinely overweight have large fat stores around their middle. However, in practice it is much easier to weigh someone than measure their waist, and so for most purposes BMI is used as an indicator of obesity.

Knowing your BMI is important, as it helps to quantify whether you are overweight or obese, and how much weight you might need to lose. It is also important in enabling your doctor or nurse to determine what type of medication would be appropriate for you, as some are better at helping weight loss than others (see Chapter 5).

8. Smoking history

We all know – even smokers know – that smoking is bad for our health. Smoking and diabetes both significantly increase the risk of heart attacks, strokes and foot problems, and so the combination is particularly harmful. Thankfully, smoking is less common now and most of my patients do not smoke. However, if you do smoke, please access the stop smoking services that are available free of charge on the NHS. Details are at https://www.nhs.uk/live-well/quit-smoking/nhs-stop-smoking-services-help-you-quit.

9. Digital retinal screening

Eye checks are important to detect the earliest signs of diabetic eye disease, which leads to abnormalities to the small blood vessels at the back of the eye. Diabetic eye disease can be managed, and even reversed, by controlling your blood glucose and blood pressure. However, the early changes do not affect eyesight, and the only way of knowing whether you have them is by having a photograph taken of your retina. In the UK we are fortunate to have a comprehensive eye-screening service, which is free of charge for people with diabetes. This is separate from the usual eye test you have to determine whether you need glasses. In many countries, the person with diabetes must arrange and pay for an eye examination (often with an eye specialist).

Digital retinal screening involves drops being put into your eyes that dilate the pupils (makes them bigger) so that the camera has a good view of the retina behind it. You will then be asked to sit still in front of a specialised camera that takes a photograph of your retina through the pupil. The image is usually ready immediately, and in many cases the person taking it will be able to show it to you. It will then be transmitted to a grading centre, where an expert will assess it for evidence of any diabetic eye disease. In due course, you will receive a letter confirming the findings. If all is well, you will be invited back for another test after one or two years. If there is evidence of retinopathy, then a further test may be recommended in six months or earlier. In the meantime, it would be good to consider what you can do to ensure your glucose levels and blood pressure are as near to normal as possible.

If the image shows evidence of more severe retinopathy, an appointment will be made for you to see an eye specialist (ophthalmologist) who can perform a more detailed examination and discuss possible treatments with you.

Meanwhile, the most important thing you can do is to turn up for your eye test. Some people have told me how fearful they are of having the test done, in case it shows some evidence of diabetic eye disease. While I can understand this perfectly natural fear, I would urge you not to let it stop you having the test done. In the early stages, good control of blood glucose levels can stop retinopathy progressing, and even help reverse it. For more advanced disease, treatment is available which can keep it under control and prevent blindness.

Getting support to manage your diabetes

The successful management of diabetes is largely down to self-management – as pretty much everything someone does can affect their blood glucose levels. This makes it so important that everyone with diabetes receives the appropriate education to teach them how best to manage the condition. Over the past twenty years there has been a huge growth in the provision of self-management education in the UK, which is something to be welcomed. In the post-pandemic era of Zoom, an increasing number of programmes can be attended remotely, which makes them even more accessible.

Most programmes are provided as weekly sessions over six to eight weeks. This may be enough to provide information, but is unlikely to help with the long-term behaviour changes that are needed to reverse the condition. Many local groups are being set up to provide this support. There is also online support available free of charge via a weekly session provided by the Public Health Collaboration. Visit https://phcuk.org/support/ for more information.

There is also high-quality information available online for people who wish to follow a low-carbohydrate approach to managing their diabetes. I recommend that my patients use the information on www.newforestpcn.co.uk/low-carb/ and the app available at https://lowcarbfreshwell.com/ – it has been accredited as a structured education programme for people with diabetes.

There are several UK-based internet forums where people can exchange information and ideas. The biggest forums are hosted by www.diabetes.co.uk and www.diabetes.org.uk (the website of the Diabetes UK charity). Although there is no guarantee that the advice given will work for everyone, or indeed that it is accurate, I have been extremely impressed with the quality of advice provided on these forums. I have no hesitation in recommending them to anyone who wishes to draw on the experience of other people with diabetes, particularly when it comes to trying out new ideas regarding diets and eating plans.

Such forums also provide an opportunity for people to share their experiences and concerns about their diabetes: there will always be someone who has had a similar experience and who has found a way through it that they are willing to share. See the Appendix for a list of useful websites.

Of course, you should never make any changes to your medication without first discussing it with your doctor or diabetes nurse.

Managing Type 2 diabetes when you are unwell

People with Type 2 diabetes are at greater risk of ill health because diabetes affects other illnesses, and other illnesses affect diabetes. The best way to minimise this effect is to ensure that your glucose levels are as near normal as possible; this book has been written to help you achieve that. But it is important to be aware that there are some situations that might make you more insulin resistant again and cause your glucose levels to increase. This section will provide you with the information you need to keep yourself as well as possible when you are ill.

As we have discussed, keeping blood glucose levels as normal as possible will help prevent further health problems, such as eye, foot or kidney disease. It will also help ensure that, if you become ill, any effect of having diabetes will be minimised. This was highlighted during the Covid-19 pandemic, when people with diabetes who had high glucose levels did less well than those with lower levels.

It is important to recognise that any illness puts a stress on the body and is associated with activation of the immune system and increased levels of stress hormones, such as cortisol and adrenaline. As I explained earlier, these hormones counter the effect of insulin and therefore increase insulin resistance, causing glucose to be released from the liver into the bloodstream. Even if your diabetes is generally under very good control, any illness can make your blood glucose levels rise. While high glucose levels for a few weeks because of illness are unlikely to lead to significant long-term damage, the high glucose may cause unpleasant symptoms as well as prolong the illness and hamper recovery, especially if you have an infection.

Even a mild viral illness, which may cause no more than a headache and a runny nose, may have a profound effect on blood glucose levels. In a similar way, people with diabetes can experience high glucose levels after a vaccination. In a sense this is a good sign, as it indicates that the vaccine has activated the immune system, but it is understandably a cause of concern, as the effect can last for a few weeks.

Whether you manage your diabetes with diet and lifestyle changes alone or with medication, I advise you to avoid sugary or high-carbohydrate foods when you are ill. I recommend that you drink plenty of plain water. Even if you do not regularly check your blood glucose, I suggest checking it at least once a day when you're ill – for example, first thing in the morning. If the level is above 8 mmol/l (140 mg/dL), you are advised to seek medical advice in case you require an increase in medication to help control your glucose levels while you are ill. This could mean increasing the dose of your existing medication or starting new medication just for the period of illness. If you are admitted to hospital, your diabetes should be monitored closely and be reviewed by a member of the diabetes team, who will be able to adjust your medication to stabilise your diabetes if necessary. Very often you will be able to return to your previous treatment before, or shortly after, going home.

Illness can also cause problems with kidney function, especially in people who have a degree of diabetic kidney disease, and this means that certain medications need to be stopped during anything other than a mild illness. As a rule, anyone who takes metformin or a SGLT2 inhibitor should stop taking it if they need to be admitted to hospital with an acute illness, or if they have any illness that causes dehydration, such as prolonged vomiting or diarrhoea, as these situations can increase the risk of your kidney function being affected or causing a metabolic disturbance: for example, affecting the acidity of the blood, which can lead to serious illness.

If you have impaired kidney function and take medication for high blood pressure, it may be advisable to stop this during periods of illness as well. It is a good idea to discuss this with your diabetes care team in advance, so that you know what to do if you become ill.

If you are on a sulfonylurea or insulin, the dose will need to be increased if your glucose levels rise; on the other hand, if your illness means you are not eating normally, these medications could make your blood glucose level fall too low. In that situation, it is very important to check your glucose levels more frequently. If your levels are falling below about 5 mmol/l (90 mg/dL), the dose of sulfonylurea or insulin will need to be decreased. In this situation, you should take medical advice on the best course of action, as it may be risky to stop one of these treatments completely. If you take any blood pressure medications, it is important to check your blood pressure if you are experiencing diarrhoea or vomiting that lasts more than a day, as you may need to reduce or stop the medication, especially if your kidney function is impaired.

Some medications for other conditions can also affect glucose control. The most important are steroids, usually taken as tablets (such as prednisolone). This is used in high doses for people who have severe flare-ups of asthma and other inflammatory conditions. If you need to take steroids, then you may also need to have insulin (or a higher dose of insulin) while you are on steroids.

There are many other tablets that can increase glucose levels. These include thiazide diuretics, beta blockers, antipsychotic drugs, statins and some antibiotics. Conversely, selective serotonin reuptake inhibitor (SSRI) antidepressants, such as sertraline and citalopram, can reduce glucose levels. I recommend that you read the leaflets that come with your medications, to find out if they could affect your glucose levels.

As a general rule, I would advise anyone with Type 2 diabetes who takes medication to discuss with their doctor what they should do with each of their medications in the event of illness. This will help you to create your own 'sick day rules' that you should keep handy, so that you can easily refer to the list if you become unwell. Table 12.2 provides an example.

Table 12.2. Sample sick day rules for someone with diabetes and taking medication.

Tablet	Dose	Taken for	If I become unwell
Metformin	500 mg twice a day	Diabetes	Stop if I have diarrhoea and vomiting
Dapagliflozin	10 mg daily	Diabetes	Stop if I have diarrhoea and vomiting
Gliclazide	40 mg daily	Diabetes	Check blood sugar levels. May need to increase dose to 80 mg (check with doctor)
Ramipril	5 mg daily	High blood pressure	Stop if I have diarrhoea and vomiting
Prednisolone	30 mg for five days	Flare-up of bronchitis	Increase gliclazide to 80 mg twice a day when taking this (check with doctor first)

Pregnancy

Pregnancy has important metabolic effects, including increasing insulin resistance in the later stages of pregnancy. Since Type 2 diabetes increasingly affects younger people, it is now not uncommon for women with Type 2 diabetes to be pregnant. If you are planning on getting pregnant, or if you are in the age group where you may become pregnant, it is important to be aware of how pregnancy might affect your diabetes and vice versa.

Pregnancy and diabetes – the key facts

- It is important to achieve stable control of your diabetes at the start of your pregnancy, and ideally before you get pregnant. This greatly reduces the risk of foetal abnormalities or other problems during your pregnancy.
- A high dose of folic acid (5 mg daily) is recommended from the time you start to try to conceive.
- Certain medications should be stopped before you become pregnant, or as soon as you find out you are pregnant. These include statins, some blood pressure medications (such as ACE inhibitors) and some diabetes medications (such as GLP1 analogues).
- It is important to check your glucose much more frequently, and to aim for fasting glucose levels below 5.3 mmol/l (95 mg/dL) and below 7.8 mmol/l (140 mg/dL) one hour, and 6.4 mmol/l (115 mg/dL) two hours after meals.
- It is likely that you will become less insulin resistant in the first few weeks, and then more insulin resistant as your pregnancy progresses. Insulin treatment is often used in the later stages of pregnancy to achieve the required glucose levels.
- Pregnancy can affect some diabetes-related complications, such as high blood pressure, kidney disease or diabetic eye disease. It is therefore important that these are monitored during pregnancy.

It is not recommended that you make a significant change to your diet during pregnancy. If you are on a low-carbohydrate diet when you become pregnant, then it is safe to continue this during pregnancy. As your pregnancy progresses, you may experience your glucose levels increasing. A gradual reduction in your carbohydrate intake may help prevent this, and reduce the need for insulin. If you are on a very low-carbohydrate ketogenic diet, then you should let your doctor or midwife know. Some experts consider a ketogenic diet to be unsafe in pregnancy, while others consider it a safe option.

Routine screening will show any ketones in your urine. This could otherwise be a cause for concern that you might not be eating enough, so it is important to tell your medical team if you are on a ketogenic diet. You can find out more about pregnancy and diabetes at https://www.diabetes.org.uk/guide-to-diabetes/life-with-diabetes/pregnancy.

Chapter 13

What to do when things don't go to plan

As we discussed in Chapter 3, managing Type 2 diabetes effectively means you will have to make changes to your lifestyle, and in particular what you eat. It is important that you can maintain these changes over the long term. This can be difficult, especially if you are surrounded by people who are eating foods that you cannot eat. This can be a particular problem if there are some foods that you crave, or that previously you have binged on. Some people do really well with managing their diabetes, then something happens to derail them. This could be a health problem, bereavement, loss of a job, moving house or family problems. These life events can cause stress, poor sleep, comfort eating or drinking more alcohol, any of which can be enough to knock a healthy person's routine. The effect of such a knock on someone with Type 2 diabetes can be more significant, especially if it disrupts their new eating plan. Sometimes, even without one of these events, people simply drift back into their old ways of eating, as they have been 'hardwired' over decades to eat in a certain way – and thus they will need to consciously change their eating behaviours once more.

Whatever the reason, if you find that your glucose levels or your weight have crept – or leapt! – back up, or you are back to eating foods that you had managed to stop, I recommend you take the following steps:

1. *Review your diet.* Write down what you are now eating, and check with the information provided in Chapter 3 to identify what foods could be causing your glucose levels to rise. Have you started eating more fruit, or sweet snacks? Or porridge or bread?
2. *Identify why your diet has changed.* This could be really easy to figure out – such as a big life event. Or is it because you have slipped back into old habits? Or have you experienced cravings for certain foods, and you now can't control these cravings? Do you feel 'addicted' to some foods?
3. *Don't beat yourself up!* Reflect on how well you have done so far.
4. *Do you feel able to get back on track?* If so, you might want to write out a plan that will reverse the changes that you have identified.

5. *If you are experiencing cravings, identify the 'trigger' foods that you crave,* and make a plan to work towards cutting them out completely.
6. *If you don't feel able to get back on track or exclude trigger foods,* try to accept that your glucose levels and weight will stay high for a while, and that you might benefit from an increase in medication to help keep them down. Book an appointment with your doctor or nurse for advice – and a prescription if needed.
7. *Once again, do not beat yourself up!* Acknowledge that these things happen, and that once you are feeling stronger, you will try to get back on track.

When you are ready to revisit your diet, think about the following points in particular:

1. *Have you started eating more fruit?* It might help to cut out fruit completely for a while, or limit yourself to a few berries each day.
2. *Have you allowed starchy foods to slip back into your routine?* Perhaps because you thought you were doing so well, you thought you could allow yourself to return to them. Or maybe eating them was so ingrained in you for so many years. If so, cut them out again.

3. *Are you sure there are no 'hidden carbs' in some of the foods you are eating?* Check things like sauces, salad dressings and tinned or ready meals.
4. *Are you still checking your blood glucose level before and two hours after one meal each day?* If you often find the level increases after eating, do you need to change some of your meals?
5. *Are you using cheese or nuts as snacks?* Remember that while these will have very little effect in raising your blood glucose level, their high fat and calorie content could be slowing down weight loss. Could you do without them for a while, or be stricter about the amount you eat?
6. *How much alcohol are you drinking?* Remember that alcohol in any form contains 'empty calories' and has a similar effect as sugar in leading to a fatty liver. That is before you consider the impact of any carbohydrate in some drinks, such as beers and ciders. Can you cut out alcohol for a while?
7. *Are you limiting sedentary time and building more walking into your daily routine?* If not, now might be a good time to do so.
8. *Are you on insulin or a sulfonylurea?* If the main problem is that you can't lose weight, but your glucose levels are okay, discuss with your doctor whether you would benefit from reducing the dose further.

Going through this list might highlight one or two changes you can make that will get you back on track. If, despite these changes, you still feel that you are stalling, then it may be worth seeing a dietitian, who can review what you are eating and provide some specific, personalised advice. Alternatively, or in addition, you may wish to consider introducing intermittent fasting into your routine, such as missing breakfast on a regular basis so that you have a sixteen-hour fast a few times a week. If you are already doing this, would you consider a twenty-four-hour fast by only eating one meal on one or two days each week?

[illegible]

Chapter 14

A healthy future awaits

Congratulations on reaching the final chapter! My aim in writing this book has been to give you the information you need to manage your Type 2 diabetes effectively, so that it does not impair your current – or future – quality of life. I know that some of the contents are quite upsetting – there are a lot of possible unpleasant consequences of having Type 2 diabetes. The aim of including this information is not to scare you, but to ensure that you are fully aware of the potential impact of Type 2 diabetes – and, most importantly, indicate what you can do to minimise the risk of those things happening.

This book focuses on the changes you can make that will have beneficial effects on your health. The most important change is to your diet. I make no apologies for talking about this in detail; in my view, it is the factor that can make the biggest difference between having Type 2 diabetes that is out of control and having Type 2 diabetes that is well managed. Unfortunately, I often see doctors and individuals with diabetes making the assumption that medication does the heavy lifting when it comes to managing glucose levels, to the extent that some doctors don't give their patients any detailed information about how they can make effective changes to manage their diabetes. This is calamitous: it is the lifestyle changes that have the most impact.

Sometimes relatively small changes can make a big difference. However, there is no one change that will work for everyone; you will need to identify the changes that work best for you. I invite you to set your own goals and your own plan for making lifestyle changes, based on the information I have provided in this book. It is completely up to you to decide which changes you wish to make, in which order and at what pace. If you're like me and you like to keep things simple, choose one or two changes you feel you can make to start with then, as you see the benefits of those changes, you should be encouraged to make more changes.

After thinking about diet, I suggest you think about how you can spend more time walking – and less time sitting down. Remember, building walking into your daily routine can have really significant benefits, and once it has become 'built in', it will become so automatic that you will stop thinking about making time to go out for a walk and will just do it!

One of the great benefits of making lifestyle changes to manage Type 2 diabetes is the possibility that you will reduce your need for medication – or even be able to stop it altogether. Remember, it is essential that you review your medications with your doctor or nurse before making significant changes to your diet, as some medications may need to be reduced or stopped (see Chapter 5 for more on this).

People who are able to come off all their diabetes medication and maintain an HbA1c of less than 48 mmol/mol (6.5 per cent) are said to be in remission. If that is your goal, you might like to read my book *How to Reverse Type 2 Diabetes and Prediabetes* for more detailed advice. Remission is not possible for everyone, especially if you have had diabetes for many years; nevertheless, adopting the changes I recommend in this book should help you lose weight, achieve lower glucose levels, and take less medication, all of which bring their own health benefits.

Remember that any improvements you achieve through lifestyle changes can also be reversed if you slip back into your old eating habits. But such setbacks are perfectly normal. If that happens to you, reread Chapter 13 of this book to help you get back on track.

I love to hear from people who have read my books, so please use the contact form on my website (https://www.thediabetesdoctor.co.uk/contact/) to let me know how you get on.

[illegible]

[illegible]

[illegible]

[illegible]

Appendix

Useful websites and further reading

www.thediabetesdoctor.co.uk – My website. It tells you all about me and my medical practice, gives details of my books, and tells you how to arrange a consultation with me. You can also get in touch to tell me how you got on after reading the book.

https://www.newforestpcn.co.uk/low-carb/ – A great collection of diabetes resources from GPs in the New Forest (my neck of the woods).

https://lowcarbfreshwell.com/resources/freshwell-app/ – A programme and an app to help you change your diet, from Freshwell GP practice in Essex.

www.thelowcarbkitchen.co.uk – A selection of delicious low-carb recipes by Emma Porter, who wrote the recipes for the *Low-Carb Diabetes Cookbook* (see below).

www.dietdoctor.com – An international website based in Sweden that has a huge amount of resources, information and recipes about using a low-carb lifestyle to improve your health.

www.diabetes.co.uk – A UK website run by a commercial company, not to be confused with the charity Diabetes UK. This organisation has long supported a low-carb approach and pioneered the low-carb eating programme. Home to many useful forums where you can get sensible advice and information from other people with diabetes.

www.diabetes.org.uk – Website of the national diabetes charity Diabetes UK. It contains a wealth of information, although I find much of its dietary information confusing. The charity sometimes seems ambivalent about low carbs, suggesting that this option is no better or worse than other approaches.

www.carbsandcals.com – Home of the famous Carbs & Cals books and app.

www.phcuk.org – The Public Health Collaboration website. It contains information about low-carb research and resources, including Dr Unwin's 'sugar infographics' and details of the Ambassadors Programme (ambassadors are representatives of the PHC in the UK. They work with GP practices to set up and run lifestyle support groups).

Books

The Low-Carb Diabetes Cookbook, David Cavan and Emma Porter (Ebury Digital, 2018) – Fantastic recipes created by a person with diabetes.

The Diabetes Weight-Loss Cookbook, Katie and Giancarlo Caldesi (Kyle Books, 2019) – Low-carb recipes to help reverse Type 2 diabetes.

Carbs & Cals Carb and Calorie Counter, Chris Cheyette and Yello Balolia (Chello Publishing, 2016) – The bible of carb counting.

Carbs & Cals World Foods: A visual guide to African, Arabic, Caribbean and South Asian foods for diabetes & weight management, Salma Mehar, et al. (Chello Publishing, 2019) – Includes foods from around the world.

The Complete Guide to Fasting by Jason Fung (Victory Belt Publishing, 2016) – A great practical guide to intermittent fasting.

The 8-week Blood Sugar Diet by Michael Mosley (Short Books Ltd, 2015) – A guide to using real food to achieve rapid weight loss on a low-calorie diet.

How to Reverse Type 2 Diabetes and Prediabetes, David Cavan (Allen & Unwin, 2024) – An effective, evidence-based approach to guide people with Type 2 diabetes and prediabetes towards a healthier future.

The 4 Pillar Plan: How to Relax, Eat, Move, Sleep Your Way to a Longer, Healthier Life, Dr Rangan Chatterjee (Penguin, 2017) – Make small changes to the four pillars (relaxation, food, movement and sleep) for better health.

Downsizing: How I lost 8 stone, reversed my diabetes and regained my health, Tom Watson (Kyle Books, 2020) – Tom describes how he took control of his diet and exercise after being diagnosed with Type 2 diabetes.

Acknowledgments

I am hugely grateful to my patients who over many years have taught me about the realities of living with Type 2 diabetes and especially the challenges caused by conventional treatments and diet advice that often seemed to make their problems worse. Special thanks to those who trusted me to guide them through a different approach, whether through seeing me in clinic or by reading one of my books.

I also acknowledge the contributions of an increasing circle of professional colleagues around the world (now too numerous to mention individually) who continue to inspire me with new understandings of Type 2 diabetes and new treatment possibilities.

I wish to thank my publishers Zoe Blanc and Anna Steadman at Hachette for inviting me to write this book and supporting me through the process, to my literary agent Jonathan Hayden for shaping my sometimes-random text into meaningful structure and to Jane Hammett for her excellent copy-editing to refine the text to produce the final version.

Index